TREACHERY BY DESIGN

Madison Shaw and Jack Wyatt Medical
Mysteries
Book 3

GARY BIRKEN M.D.

Erupen Titles

For Frank V. Sacco, his spirit and fortitude live on in all of us.

Part I

Chapter 1

It was pure greed that drove Roy and Paul Fergus to habitually ignore the law. Even though they were only fraternal twins, they'd grown up sharing the same gunmetal blue eyes, stocky frames, and remarkable gift of gab. From grade school to grad school, their interests and pursuits had been one and the same. Their many accomplishments were undeniable, although generally checkered with an assortment of crafty shortcuts and subtle deceptions.

It was a gusty and overcast fall day, and they had spent most of it hiking and fishing. It was nearing five o'clock when they arrived back at their secluded white-cedar cabin located in a rustic area of Southeast Virginia. Seven years ago they had earned master's degrees in engineering from the University of Illinois. Marsh Technologies, the third-largest defense contractor in the country, offered them each a position as a marine engineer in their nuclear submarine division. They'd accepted eagerly and moved to Newport News, Virginia. Confirmed bachelors and avid outdoorsmen, they'd purchased the seventy-five-year-old log cabin two years after they arrived.

After cleaning up, they stopped in the great room where Paul grabbed a couple of double-walled whiskey glasses from the Brunswick-style bar and poured them each two ounces of their favorite ten-year-old bourbon. After clinking their glasses together, they strolled out onto the covered porch where they grabbed seats in matching wicker rockers to wait for the aloof man they knew only as Andrey. For the past two years, on the third Saturday of every month, they'd met him on the porch at exactly at five-fifteen p.m.

"What time do you think he'll be here?" Paul asked.

Looking at his brother through dubious eyes with a face bathed in annoyance, Roy responded, "We've been meeting with this guy every month on the same day and at the same time for the past two years. He's never been late yet. Does that fact help you answer your own question?"

"I'm just making conversation. Try not to be such a jerk," Paul said, trying to control a temper that flared far too often.

While they chatted about their day's activities and a frustrating problem with their latest project at work, they kept their eyes trained on the single-lane dirt road that gave access to the cabin. The twins knew from experience that Andrey would be arriving on foot. He never parked near the cabin, prompting them to assume it was his preference to keep the make, license plate, and any other identifying features of his car confidential.

Roy gave his brother two quick taps on the shoulder. "There he is."

"I wonder how many meetings like this he has a week?"

"Who cares? Try and keep your eye on the ball."

"What's that supposed to mean?"

"It means don't let your curiosity get the best of you. We have a business relationship with this guy, and that's where it ends. I don't care if he's a trust-fund baby, a bridge tender, or a professional saxophone player, nor could I care less what business he conducts when he's not standing in front of us."

"So he doesn't worry you at all?"

"I didn't say that. But for the last two years, we've had an enormously profitable relationship with him, and unless you know something I don't, he's always been square with us. Beyond that, nothing matters to me."

"Excuse me for being so cautious but I believe in keeping your friends close and your mysterious business associates closer."

Roy's eyes tightened, but he couldn't hold back a grin. "You're hopeless."

As Andrey approached, they noticed his gaze was fixed on them. He walked with the same broad-based gait they'd observed the first time they met him. As he always did, he wore aviator-style sunglasses despite the fading light and a washed-out red baseball cap tipped slightly to the right. He had an unsmiling face, a wiry physique, and a full head of coarse, prematurely gray hair. From what little they'd learned of him from their brief meetings, he seemed to have the patience of a stray cat with a kidney stone.

"Do you have it?" he asked, as he ascended the recently painted porch steps.

"Right here," Roy said, handing him a large, tape-sealed manila envelope.

"I'll see you in four weeks," he said, tossing a bulky white envelope in their direction that Roy caught with one hand.

"There are a couple of things we should discuss," Paul said.

Andrey stopped on the steps, looking annoyed. He and swung his gaze toward him. "You'll be informed when I feel it's time for a chat."

"And if that's not acceptable to us?"

Going silent for a moment, Andrey removed his sunglasses. "I've never considered you a towering intellectual, so I'm going to make this as clear as I can for you. I've made you and your brother very rich men. Don't get too smart with me, Paul; I'm pretty smart myself. It could end badly for you. Take a lesson from your brother, who seems to understand the importance of keeping his mouth shut."

Fearing Paul's conversation with Andrey was on the brink of erupting into something beyond unpleasant, Roy laid a cautionary hand on his brother's forearm. "We look forward to seeing you in a month." Without uttering another syllable, Andrey straightened his cap, descended the last two steps, and started back down the road without so much as a backward glance. As soon as he was out of earshot, Roy turned to his brother. "For god's sake, are you trying to get us killed?"

"You were always the more politically correct one of us. Obviously, he doesn't scare me the way he scares you. There's a time for charming the birds out of the trees and a time for hard-nosed business tactics. I'm unconvinced you know the difference."

"I told you the same thing last month and the month before; when the time's right, we'll hit him up for more money."

A subdued grin landed on Paul's face. "Sometimes I think you forget that, without us, Andrey and whomever he's working with could close up shop."

Growing more impatient by the minute with his brother's obstinance, Roy finger-combed his hair and stood up.

"Talking to you is about as helpful as watering a dead flower. C'mon. Let's go inside and pan fry some of those brown bass."

Chapter 2

After finishing their dinner, Roy and Paul built a blazing fire in their natural-stone fireplace, drank a generous amount of brandy from crystal snifters, and began a best-of-three chess match. When it reached eleven p.m., they were well inebriated and in the middle of the third game. Deciding to call it a night, they left the board intact with the intention of picking up where they'd left off at a later time and headed off to their respective bedrooms. Compounding the excessive brandy they'd consumed, they were both naturally heavy sleepers.

At ten minutes past two in the morning, a woman dressed in a navy-blue sweat suit with a fanny pack around her waist silently climbed the porch stairs. She was just under six feet tall and well toned from her intense daily workout. In her fanny pack she carried a small flashlight, a screwdriver, a unique lightbulb, and a Glock 26 semiautomatic handgun.

This morning's visit was her second covert trip to the Ferguses' cabin. The first was three days earlier when Roy and Paul were in Newport News working an eighteen-hour day. Their busy schedule left her undisturbed as she thoroughly surveyed both the interior and exterior of the cabin. What she'd learned became the framework for the plan that she would execute in less than an hour. Beyond this one operation, there were no other requirements to fulfill her lucrative contract.

Having limited concerns that anybody was likely to break in to their cabin, the Ferguses had never replaced the simple lock that secured the front door. It was the same one that was in place the day they'd moved in. Based on her experience of easily picking the lock the first time she'd visited, she anticipated no problem gaining access to the cabin now. Her gut feeling was correct, and a minute after she began working the lock, she was standing in the entranceway. Before moving any farther into the cabin, she spent a minute leaning against a walnut storage chest with her ears perked for any sound that either of the Fergus twins was awake. After a time, she moved out of the entranceway and headed into the great room.

She removed the flashlight from her fanny pack and made her way over to a tan leather couch with matching solid wood end tables. Atop the table on the left sat a simple lamp that the Ferguses had connected to a timer that triggered the lights to come on at six p.m. on the nights the cabin was unoccupied. Wasting no time, she reset the timer to turn the light on in precisely thirty minutes. She then tilted the lampshade back, unscrewed the sixty-watt bulb, and replaced it with the one she'd brought with her. Earlier in the day, she'd used a tiny drill bit to create an opening in the bulb just large enough for her to insert a hypodermic needle. Using a ten-cc syringe, she'd filled the bulb halfway with gasoline. When she was finished, she'd patched the opening with wax.

When she was satisfied with her makeshift detonator, she moved into the kitchen. Against the back wall stood a white antique gas stove that the prior owner had told Paul and Roy was part of the original construction in the late 1950s. On her first visit, she'd noted that the natural gas line was showing signs of significant corrosion. Taking a couple of steps closer to the stove, she kneeled down and removed the screwdriver from her fanny pack. She pushed its tip into the area of the most severe corrosion, the tool easily penetrating the damaged line, creating a sizable gas leak. She pressed on, pushing and rotating the tool until she had extended the opening by another inch.

Coming out of her kneeling position, she made her way back through the great room and exited the cabin the same way she'd come in. Her total time inside was eleven minutes.

It was a windswept morning, and as she descended the porch steps, she inhaled a lungful of the damp, chilly air. It took her six minutes to make the walk back to the SUV she'd rented under a fictitious name. Climbing onto the hood of the vehicle, she leaned back against the windshield. She estimated she was a quarter of a mile from the cabin. She raised her eyes and briefly stared up at the magnificent Beaver Moon. After a few minutes, she checked the time again. It was two forty-two.

Three minutes later, the light in Roy and Paul's great room came on. In a matter of a few seconds, the filament ignited the gasoline. The flame grew rapidly, shattering the glass bulb. The blast of the massive explosion rocked the tranquil night air. The sky itself seemed to detonate with a towering burst of saw-toothed, luminous flames partially hidden beneath plumes of gray-white smoke that stretched high above the tree line. Mixed together with the flames and smoke, thousands of cabin fragments were blown into the night sky as if they'd been captured by the full force of a tornado.

The woman felt the hood beneath her shudder as the windshield rattled from the explosion's powerful shock wave. After watching for a few more seconds, she slid off the front of the SUV, walked back to the driver's-side door, opened it, and got in. She had no doubt the Fergus twins had perished in the explosion. A minute later, she was on her way home.

She viewed herself as a person who wasn't easily impressed with her accomplishments, but this morning was the rare exception. The spectacle of the cabin explosion and the exhilaration she'd felt watching her plan come to fruition with geometric precision made her spirits soar like nothing else she'd ever experienced.

Chapter 3

FOURTEEN MONTHS LATER WASHINGTON, D.C.

Walking with purpose down Pennsylvania Avenue, John Winkler's mind was filled with trepidation regarding his impending meeting. An engineer in the ship-building division at Marsh Technologies, he had finally gathered the courage to request a meeting with Oren Severin, the vice president he reported to, to discuss a matter of grave importance that John believed posed a threat to national security. He'd implored Severin to dismiss the standard corporate protocol and agree to meet with him at an off-campus location. Based on their long professional relationship, Oren had agreed to the request by convincing himself he wasn't stepping over a line— he was just moving it slightly.

The two men had begun their careers at Marsh within a few months of each other, but they'd each taken a different course. Oren, being the more driven and politically adept of the two, climbed the corporate ladder with greater speed than John. After thirteen years, his meteoric career landed him a place in Marsh's C-suite. In contrast, as the months led to years, John, who had never been particularly ambitious, remained content to advance slowly in the organization. The intellectual challenges of his job and the compensation package met all his needs.

The day the CEO announced Oren had been named vice president, John couldn't have been happier for him and was the first one at his door to congratulate him on the promotion. Much of John's effectiveness as an engineer was fueled by an uncanny grasp of computer technology. It was a talent powered by equal parts remarkable aptitude and a healthy dose of God-given talent.

Holding a large white envelope tightly in his hand, John strolled past Freedom Plaza and entered Pershing Park. The greenspace, named for the celebrated General John J. Pershing, spanned nearly two acres and consisted of stately trees, picturesque gardens, and several displays honoring the United States' contribution to winning World War I. John made his way over to a long bench that faced a stern-faced bronze statue of the general with his field glasses in hand. In stark contrast, John was a small-chinned, scrawny man with small, unblinking hazel eyes. His daily five o'clock shadow seemed as much a part of his natural facial features as the chin and cheeks it covered.

Nervously checking the time, he coaxed his rimless sunglasses a bit farther down on the bridge of his concave nose. Feeling the strap muscles of his neck stiffen, he exhaled a weighted breath from the deepest part of his lungs. He took a hasty look around, craning his neck to the right and then back to the left. He then stared beyond the park, training his eyes on the Washington Monument. Despite his self-warnings to stay calm, John's gut knotted with angst that sent a wave of nausea across his upper abdomen.

He tried to distract himself with reassurances that what he believed he'd discovered was not only irrefutable but of major importance. Whether the powers that be at Marsh would take him seriously was anybody's guess, and he hoped Oren would be able to find out. In the worst-case scenario, they could share in a belly laugh and consider his theory to be the work of a fanciful imagination.

Despite the fact that his intentions were genuine, Marsh's elite might take a dim view of him exploring a company matter that was not only outside his scope of work but very possibly above his security clearance. It suddenly dawned on him that continuing to worry and second-guess his decision to set up the meeting with Oren served no useful purpose. He'd made his decision, and he pushed away any further thoughts of calling it off while there was still time.

He watched as two young women wearing George Washington University sweatshirts rollerbladed by. When he glanced back toward the entrance, he spotted Oren coming toward him. With his usual genial face, he approached with a slight limp, a constant reminder of his glory days as a college lacrosse player at Gettysburg College. He took the seat next to John and extended his hand.

"It's good to see you," John said.

"You as well. Suzie sends her regards."

"Please share my fondest regards with her as well. Annette mentioned to me that she'd spoken with Suzy last week —something about going to a lecture at American University in early December."

"So, what's up? You sounded more than a little anxious when you called," Oren said in his quintessential Irish brogue, a product of spending the first fourteen years of his life residing in a small village on the west coast of Kerry County. "I don't get invited to a lot of cloak-and-dagger meetings, so I can't wait to find out what's on your mind," he added, rubbing his palms together.

John took a few moments to collect himself before beginning. "I came across something I'm concerned about that I'd like to share with you. Maybe I'm jumping to conclusions, or my imagination's running away with me, but before doing something dumb, I wanted to get your opinion on whether you think I should inform the company or not."

Oren laid his arm on the back of the bench. "I know we go back a long way, so I hope you take what I'm about to say in the spirit it's intended."

"Of course."

"Before you get started, are you sure this isn't something that you'd prefer to pursue through normal channels." He held up a quieting hand. "I mention this only to make sure that you realize that once you share this information with me, it might become a very tough bell to unring."

"I've thought about all that and I'm certain this is the way I'd like to handle the problem. It's a complicated situation, and there are parts of what I've discovered that I suspect are well above my pay grade." John handed him the envelope absent any hesitation. "I put the whole thing together in a report. If, after reading it, you want to take it up the chain of command… Well, I'll leave that decision up to you. If you think it belongs in the trash, I'm okay with that as well."

Nodding slowly, Oren responded, "I'll be happy to take a look at your report, but I don't want to assume the role of the all-seeing arbitrator. After I read it, I think we should discuss it and make a decision as to the best way to manage things."

"I'm fine with that as well. The only request I'd like to make is that, for now, I'd appreciate it if you'd consider my report for your eyes only."

"I can do that for now, but I can't promise I'll be able to sit on it if I feel it contains information that has to be kicked upstairs and you suddenly decide that's not what you want to do." A cautionary look took form on Oren's face. "I'm sure you understand that if you've come across something of critical importance and we cover it up…well, in a flicker of an eye we could both wind up in a gated community making license plates."

John shared in Oren's amusement with a fleeting chuckle. "The thought of that hadn't crossed my mind, but maybe it should have."

"You know, John, there are many of us at Marsh who are well aware you're a magician when it comes to computer technology. I hope you didn't take too many liberties when you embarked on this quest of yours."

"I thought you might mention that, and if it's okay with you, I'd rather save that conversation until after you've read my report."

"I suspect you already know there've been times when we've turned a blind eye to your expert computer skills because of the outstanding job you do and your value to the company."

"I'd be the first to admit that I can be a little unconventional at times, but sometimes it's easier for me to be creative about the ways I gather information that's critical to my work. It's a lot more efficient and beats the hell out of waiting three weeks to get the data from a reluctant employee when I can get it myself before lunch any day of the week."

"While I appreciate your devotion to your job, count yourself among the fortunate that you haven't suffered any adverse consequences from your unique methods. The day may come that you'll regret having taken such a casual view of Marsh's policies and procedures."

"I love my job, Oren, and I'd hate to be told to clean out my locker and turn in my ID. I wouldn't have put you in this difficult situation if I thought this was something minor."

"I think we're getting a little off the topic. As soon as I've had a chance to read your report, I'll give you a call."

"I don't mean to sound pushy, but when can I expect to hear from you?"

"You may not have meant it, but that definitely sounded pushy," Oren said, rubbing the envelope between his thumb and index finger. "This doesn't feel too thick. Do you think I can get through it in...say thirty minutes?"

"I think so."

"In that case, why don't you take a couple of spins around the park, and I'll read your report right now?"

"Thanks for not making me suggest that. I'll be back in thirty minutes," he said, getting to his feet and quickly walking away before Oren changed his mind.

Chapter 4

John's time estimate was accurate. After thirty minutes, Oren had thoroughly read the report and had no trouble deciding it was far too credible and important to feed into the shredder. It was typical of John's work product: logical, highly organized, and persuasive. Lifting his eyes from the pages, he noticed the temperature had dropped several degrees, the wind had kicked up, and the picture-perfect sky now contained a gathering of thick gray rain clouds.

"What do you think?" came a voice from behind him as John came around the bench and retook his seat.

Oren held up the report for emphasis. "I'll be honest with you. I don't quite know what to think. If there's any chance your theory's correct...well, we've got one hell of a problem on our hands."

"I can't speak to all the possible consequences, but I'm pretty close to convinced the material in my report is accurate."

"You realize you're suggesting there's been an intentional and material breach of national security that's gone undetected."

"I'm fully aware of that. So where do we go from here?"

"That's the easy part. It's not our job to be the judge and jury in these types of matters. But it is our responsibility to report a possible infraction like this to the Defense Contract Management Agency."

Cautious in his choice of words, John said, "I assumed, if you thought it was necessary to pursue the matter, you'd begin by taking my report to Marsh's C-suite, not the DCMA."

"And under normal circumstances, you'd be right," he said with all honesty. "But for reasons I'd prefer not to get into, informing our team first may not be the best way to handle this particular situation."

John's face became bathed with worry. "You realize you'd be going way outside the prescribed chain of command?"

"I do."

"Are you hearing me? You could lose your job."

Oren nodded deliberately. "Quite easily, I expect."

"Just how do you plan to proceed?"

"I haven't quite worked that out yet," he said, putting his hand on John's shoulder. "But it might be better for now if you left this to me. You did the right thing bringing your concerns to the company's attention."

"What is it that you're not saying?"

"You've met your responsibility, and you should leave the rest to me." From the look in his eyes, it was clear to John he was trying to protect him.

Unable to keep a straight thought in his head, John asked him directly, "Can I expect to ever hear from you again about this matter?"

Oren came to his feet, extended his hand, and said, "I don't have the first damn clue, but I appreciate you having the trust and confidence in our relationship to bring this situation to my attention."

A puzzled look remained on John's face as he shook Oren's hand. With nothing further to be said, he turned and headed toward the exit. Any doubts he'd had about being taken seriously had evaporated. But he didn't feel the wave of relief that he'd thought he would. To the contrary; all at once, he feared his insistence upon meeting with Oren might turn out to be the most regrettable mistake of his life.

Chapter 5

While John was making his way to the park's exit, Oren decided to take a stroll to give himself a few more minutes to ponder the predicament John had just presented him with. After a time, he came across an isolated bench and sat down. Oren was an intuitive man, well schooled in the realities of the corporate culture. Marsh Technologies was in the business of fulfilling big-ticket government contracts. Sometimes, when an unexpected and dicey problem arose, their modus operandi was to provide the most expeditious solution and damage control. The price for that approach was that integrity and disclosure oftentimes got lost in the shuffle. Oren was a decent man who knew how to do the right thing. He also knew how to handle himself in the prickly Marsh corporate culture. It was doing them both at the same time that kept him struggling.

Finally, after listening to his inner voice, he came to realize two things were certain: First, he knew what he had to do. Second, he didn't have the luxury of time to try and convince himself he was right. For a few moments he gazed around at his surroundings. He remained surprised John hadn't grasped the obvious advantage of bypassing the Marsh leadership and going directly to the DCMA.

Dismissing what he'd promised John a short fifteen minutes ago, Oren reached for his phone and placed a call.

"Defense Contract Management Agency. How may I help you?"

"Please connect me to the office of Mr. Ed Terry," he said, bolstering his conviction with every word he uttered.

"This is Ed Terry."

"Hi, Ed. It's Oren Severin."

"It's always nice hearing from you, but I thought our meeting wasn't until next week."

"I'm afraid I may have come across something regarding a couple of our contracts that could be problematic. I'm not comfortable waiting until next week to brief you. If you can find some time sooner, I think we should talk."

"Of course. And if you don't mind me saying so, you sound beyond concerned. I'm free now if you'd like to discuss the matter on the phone."

"Before I get into the nuts and bolts of this thing, I'd like to ask you a question."

"Shoot."

"I understand there's a reporting pathway I can avail myself of that guarantees me anonymity."

"That's correct, but you're dealing with the government, and sometimes strict policies don't always convert to reality. But listen, we've known each other a long time, and if you feel remaining anonymous is essential, I'll do everything in my power to make it happen." Ed had been encouraging but had left the door open a crack. It was what Oren expected and a conditional promise he was ready to accept.

"Coming from you, that's good enough for me. But if you don't mind, I'd rather not talk about this on the phone."

"I understand."

"When are you available to meet?"

"I don't know," Ed responded in a nonchalant voice. "How long will it take you to get over to my office?"

Chapter 6

ONE WEEK LATER

Everett Warren, the chairman of the board of Marsh Technologies, often bragged he'd never suffered a failed dream. Pot-bellied, with two discolored moles on the chin of his all-too-often sour face, he appeared considerably older than his fifty-three years. Possessed with unbridled ambition and vision, he'd brought Marsh Technologies to higher plateaus than any other board chairman had in the company's fifty-eight-year history. Entirely comfortable in his own skin, the only flaw he'd admit to was his incurable weakness for material possessions. Making the short list of his most coveted belongings was his one-year-old emerald green Maybach limousine.

Sitting comfortably in the back seat, Everett gazed out the window as Claude, his chauffer for the past ten years, proceeded slowly down Constitution Avenue. Heavy on his mind was the distinct possibility that he was about five minutes away from attending a meeting that could prove to be the most consequential of his career. Marsh was in the throes of a crisis, and Everett was well aware that righting the ship would be a delicate and challenging task. Handled improperly, the company could very rapidly become a faint memory as one of the country's major defense contractors.

"That's him with the blue umbrella. Pull over," he told Claude, as the Maybach approached the Herbert C. Hoover building. Once he parked at the curb, Claude exited the limo, walked around to the curbside door, and opened it for James Brubaker, a tall man with a black circle beard and angular shoulders.

Everett had never met him in person but had spoken to him on the phone on two occasions over the past few days. He didn't strike Everett as a stand-alone genius, but he did seem articulate and clearly focused on the problem at hand. From what little he knew of him, Brubaker viewed him as similar to many of the individuals he'd met over the years who'd made their careers in government.

While Brubaker settled in, he took a few seconds to have a thorough look around and examine the polished brass trim.

"You're six minutes late," he said, as he continued to study the interior of the limousine.

"We hit a little more traffic than we expected."

"It's nice to meet you face to face," Brubaker stated. "I've read a lot about you in a number of different business journals. I'm sorry I requested this meeting on such short notice, but we're facing a calamitous situation, and time is of the essence. Unfortunately, we're clearly dealing with something that I'm afraid was handled rather poorly right from the beginning."

"I won't disagree with that, but I'm optimistic we can focus on the present and find a solution to the problem."

"Your optimism is commendable. As we used to say in the military, when you find yourself overrun by overwhelming forces—don't retreat, reload."

"I couldn't agree more," Everett said, having served in the Army as an infantry officer and being quite familiar with the expression. "You mentioned on the phone that you'd be able to provide me with a general idea of how we might approach things."

"Normally, our position would be to stay clear of something like this and let your organization sort things out on your own. But because of the potential embarrassment to some rather key people, we're going to help you out." He extended his legs and crossed them at the ankles. "You know, Everett, it didn't help that Marsh wasn't exactly forth-coming about the problem." With a cynical grin he added, "If it weren't for the Defense Contract Management Agency's anonymous reporting policy, we might still be in the dark about things."

"With all due respect, we just found out about the report ourselves."

"Let's not quibble about it. I've been a longtime believer that people's erroneous confidence in reporting things confidentially has to be one of our best forms of intelligence gathering."

"Obviously, in retrospect, we understand we could have handled things a lot better."

"It's not exactly a *we* now, is it? But I admire you taking the *buck stops here* approach. I guess all mega-corporations have had to deal with a renegade employee from time to time. I think we passed the blame exit about fifty miles back. There's no reason to dwell on mistakes and bad judgment. What I'm here to tell you is that efforts are under way to correct matters, and what we need is Marsh's complete cooperation and discretion until the matter's taken care of."

"Were on the same page—you needn't worry about a thing," Everett assured him.

"You'll forgive me for saying this, but I get paid to worry about things people tell me not to worry about." Everett fiddled with his gold cufflink. He felt Brubaker's watchful eyes moving across his face. "Here's how we're going to do this—you'll be contacted by one of our freelance consultants who we utilize from time to time, strictly on a contract basis. To a person, they're totally non-political and non-partisan. They don't question our motives, and we don't question their methods. It's always been a productive working rela-tionship. We'll need one resource person at Marsh to provide us with detailed updates as things start to unwind. Obviously, that can't be you. We've heard good things about your CEO. He might be a good choice, but whoever you pick, only give that person as much information as they need. Remember, discretion is the coin of the realm."

"Understood. I'll brief Erik Brickell today."

"Make sure he's clear on what we expect of him. He's to play a supportive role. The freelancer we'll use won't require his direct help in any way. Understood?"

"Perfectly."

"Good. You can let me out right up there…and I can open the door myself." Warren tapped on the glass partition and Claude pulled up to the curb. "There's no reason for us to speak again. We'll be watching from afar. We're not talking about a minor flesh wound here, Everett. If we don't handle this thing just right, it's quite possible there won't be enough parachutes to go around."

"Do you have any idea when things may start to take form?"

"They already have," he said, as he stepped out of the Maybach.

Everett drew in a large breath and held it for a few moments before allowing it to slip between his lips. He glanced through his window at the glacial pace of the morning traffic. He felt a slight quiver in his fingertips that quickly traveled up to his wrists. He couldn't help but wonder what the future could possibly hold in store for him.

He grimaced inwardly with the realization that public humiliation and jail time were remote but real possibilities.

———

WALKING WEST ON CONSTITUTION AVENUE, Brubaker knew the president's chief of staff, Hammett Jones, was anxiously awaiting his call. Prior to making that call, he wanted to take a few minutes to further ponder his conversation with Warren and how best to present what he learned to Jones. He continued to walk at a brisk pace. After a brief time, he glanced around, reached for his phone, and placed the call. Jones answered on the first ring.

"Good morning, Bru. How did it go?"

"I'm pleased with the results, sir. Mr. Warren clearly understands the situation and is prepared to do whatever's necessary to make the problem go away."

"That's good to hear. How much of an understanding does he have of the delicacy of the situation?"

"Based on his highly cooperative attitude, I didn't feel it was necessary to provide him with specific details. With that said, I can assure you he has a full understanding that the government's position is that the security level of this situation should be considered top secret."

"You sound certain in your assessment."

"I am, sir. Warren was very forthcoming about his overwhelming desire to get this problem in Marsh's rear-view mirror as quickly and quietly as possible."

"Needless to say, the old man isn't too pleased about this unexpected problem. He was under the impression that this problem had been taken care of long ago. He's got one term left before spending the rest of his days fly fishing back home in Idaho and writing his memoirs. A messy scandal's not exactly what he has in mind for his swan song. He wants the problem dealt with, and he doesn't want to hear another word about it. I don't have to remind you that we both serve at his pleasure."

"I fully intend to make sure the president's plans for his retirement come to fruition in a seamless manner."

"I'm glad to hear you say that, although I've never doubted your affection and loyalty for him. Please keep me advised."

Brubaker returned his phone to its case and continued walking toward the President's Park South. He had spent many years in government service dealing with and solving demanding problems. Risky and sensitive situations had never deterred him from doing what needed to be done. He had no reason to suspect that effectively dealing with Marsh Technologies' problem would be any different.

Chapter 7

FIVE DAYS LATER

In a way, Regan Cullen had made peace with herself long ago about her chosen profession. She'd reached a point where going from one day to the next without ever being hampered by regret or remorse had become second nature to her. With long Verona-brown hair, a flawless complexion, and low cheekbones, she carried herself with confidence. At thirty-two years of age, she had become an effective freelancer with a rare skill set. It was an unorthodox way to pay her bills, but it provided her with an extremely comfortable lifestyle.

She viewed safeguarding her fellow citizens' freedoms not as a job—but as her calling. Her methods were oftentimes dangerous and brutal, but for her, they were professional imperatives where the end always justified the means. She'd never been inclined to consider the moral implications of what her job demanded. She believed the average citizen had an unshakable expectation that it was the government's sworn responsibility to protect their safety and freedom—the manner in which they provided this blanket of protection mattered little to them.

After she'd gotten out of the military, Regan had had no preference as to where she'd settle down. She'd simply assumed her job would dictate the location, which was exactly the way it turned out. The person she was closest to in the world was her older brother. He was ex-military and currently working as an agent in the Bureau of Diplomatic Security. He suspected how his sister made her living, but he thought it better, for a host of reasons, to blindly accept her cover story that she was a director of IT for a small company.

For her current assignment, she had been engaged in the usual way—a phone call followed by an encrypted email that provided her all the information and resources she'd need. The rules of the unwritten contract were simple: Failure was never an option, and the first time she turned down an operation would be the last one she'd ever be offered. Her current assignment had come to her attention two days ago and allowed her three days to plan and begin moving the initiative forward.

After her third fourteen-hour day organizing every detail and considering every conceivable misstep of the operation, Regan entered the employee's entrance to the one-hundred-fifty-eight-thousand-square-foot corporate headquarters of Marsh Technologies Incorporated. It was one a.m.

Wearing a long-sleeved teal-colored shirt displaying the company's purple hexagonal logo and black cargo pants, she paused to clock in using her perfectly forged employee ID. She then made her way along the back corridor until she reached the stairwell, where she went down a single flight of stairs to the Department of Office Inventory Management, which was the organization's hub for distributing all manner of office supplies.

The expansive area was dimly lit. The subtle scent of peppermint created by the sophisticated odor-diffusing system floated in the air. Having been briefed by knowledgeable sources and having diligently studied the blueprints of the building, Regan made her way to station twenty-two of the assembly section, where dozens of well-stocked carts were ready to be taken out on delivery. Even though the staff on the night shift was minimal, Regan scanned the area carefully. When she saw nobody, she moved in behind her cart and wheeled it toward the elevators.

Without a scintilla of nervousness, she boarded the elevator and rode it up to the ninth floor. She had only taken a few steps down the faintly lit hallway when she first noticed the silhouette of an approaching man. Taking the unexpected situation in stride, Regan continued toward him as if her presence was nothing out of the ordinary. When he was about fifteen feet away, she recognized the hulking figure as a security guard. He had pock-marked skin and a courteous smile.

"Morning," he said, hooking his thumbs around the top edge of his black duty belt.

"Hi," she responded, noting that he was unarmed and a bit on the slovenly side for a security guard. She watched as his gaze centered on her ID badge.

"I haven't seen you before, Kathleen."

"I'm part of the relief team. Claudia's still sick, so they assigned me to cover her deliveries. My schedule's pretty unpredictable, so that's probably why we've never met."

"So you don't have a regular route?"

"Nope. We provide back-up wherever we're needed. We have over fifty of us on the team. Somebody's always getting sick or on vacation, so we have a separate call schedule to cover their routes whenever necessary."

"Do you like it better than having a regular route?"

With an indifferent shrug, she responded, "I can't say I've given it much thought. But I'll tell you one thing, it kind of cuts down on the monotony."

"I've been here a while and you're the first sub I've run into. There must be a better way."

"Well, if you can come up with a system to keep all these folks stocked up and happy when it comes to their supplies, I'm sure the head of Inventory Management would love to talk to you about it." She slowly moved her cart forward, hoping he'd get the hint she had better things to do than chat with him. "One thing about Marsh, if you come up with a great idea, there's usually something extra in your pay envelope come Christmas."

"What a nice surprise that would be," he told her with a wink. "Have a nice holiday season."

"The same to you," she said with a casual wave, pleased with her facility in dealing with the inquisitive security guard's unexpected appearance. As soon as he was out of sight, Regan wheeled the cart down the central hallway toward her first stop on a prearranged route that would take her to several floors. Once more, she checked the time. She'd lost a few minutes dealing with the talkative guard, but she was sure it wouldn't impact significantly on the time she'd projected to finish the task at hand.

An hour later she had made her last stop. Returning to the basement level, she replaced the cart in its designated slot and exited the building as if she had just completed another humdrum shift at work.

Taking a deep breath of the damp morning air, she detected the subtle scent of ozone that persisted from an earlier shower. She made the six-block walk to her parked car, and twenty minutes later, she slipped the latchkey into the front door of her condominium. As he walked into her entranceway, she couldn't contain a mammoth yawn. Knowing she was about ten minutes away from climbing into bed and making up for a lot of lost sleep pleased her to no end.

Chapter 8

EIGHT DAYS LATER

Nicole Dantec Wyatt had always prided herself on her stoicism and her perpetual state of excellent health. That all came to an end earlier in the week when, at the age of forty-one, she'd contracted an illness that severely tested her emotional and physical mettle. She hadn't felt this sick since battling a nasty case of mononucleosis during her junior year of economics studies at the University of Paris. Much to her dismay, with each passing day she showed no signs of recovering.

It was a few minutes past noon, and despite having asked her seventeen-year-old daughter, Anise, to set the bedroom thermostat to seventy-six, she was still plagued by chills, light-headedness, and a serious weakness of her arms and legs. Lying semi-reclined in bed, she gathered every particle of strength she could muster and pushed herself a little higher up against the leather headboard. The energy she expended left her air hungry and worsened the relentless pulsatile headache trapped behind her right eye that radiated to her temple like the arc of a stun gun.

Nicole closed her eyes briefly, but when it felt as if the bed were spinning, she snapped them open. As she took one labored breath after another, the bone-chilling terror that she had contracted an illness more severe than she'd ever imagined suddenly consumed her again.

Feeling her anxiety nearing its red line, she called out to Anise that she needed her to come to the bedroom right away. When there was no response, Nicole repeated her plea. It was only after her third call for assistance went unanswered that she remembered Anise had told her she was running out to get some groceries and that she'd be back in an hour or so. Unfortunately, Nicole had no recollection of when Anise had left their condominium and therefore no clue as to when she'd return.

She reached a tremulous hand toward the nightstand to find her cell phone. When she realized it wasn't there, she craned her neck in both directions, desperately scanning the bedroom, hoping to spot it. Having no recollection when or where she'd used it last, she continued to look around the room—but it was to no avail. Struggling to gather herself, she rolled her comforter off her abdomen and toward her ankles.

The pain in her legs had become progressively worse over the last three days, making it challenging for her to hang them partially off the side of the bed. But she persisted, and after another few seconds, she was finally able to bring herself to a seated position. She was intent on getting up, but before attempting to come to her feet, she held her head as steady as possible for a minute to minimize the vertigo that never seemed to improve.

Nicole tried gluing her gaze on a serigraph of a beachside sunrise. She couldn't completely shake the sensation of spinning, but over the next couple of minutes she felt her sense of balance improve. With renewed optimism, she finally planted her feet squarely on the floor.

To her delight, with deep concentration, she finally managed to stand up. Allowing herself one quick mental pat on the back, she took her first guarded step. Carefully, she continued with one step at a time until she gradually made her way out of the bedroom and into the smartly decorated living room.

Being an avid marathoner and badminton player, Nicole was unaccustomed to the necessity of moving at a glacial pace to maintain her balance and avoid falling. As she approached the center of the room, she shifted her gaze to her prized black baby grand piano. She paused, holding on to the back of the leather sectional sofa to rest and steady herself. To her relief, she spotted her phone sitting on the piano's music rack. With her impatient side trumping her cautious one, she took two impulsive steps toward the piano. With one foot forward into the third step, she suddenly found herself weak-kneed and wobbly.

Instantly consumed with trepidation and fearing she was moments from falling, she extended a flailing hand and lunged toward the baby grand, praying she could save herself by grabbing hold of the lid. But shooting her hand out eliminated whatever balance she clung to and sent her toppling forward. With her tumbling body seeming to have a mind of its own, her fingertips barely reached the lid's edge. Unable to grab hold, Nicole fell to the teak floor. Her right shoulder impacted first, absorbing the brunt of the force. It was only by the slimmest of margins that she escaped a devastating blow to her head. Her body came to rest in a twisted position with one side of her face pushed flush against the floor and her right arm trapped under her torso.

Panicked to her core, it took her a minute to slow her breathing and collect herself. Her shoulder ached, and it took every ounce of strength she could muster to free her arm from its pinned position beneath her. Her eyes darted from one side of the room to the other looking for the closest piece of furniture she could use to help boost herself up. The only promising option was the piano bench. If she could manage to get to it, there was a chance she could hoist herself up enough to reach her phone and call for help.

Once again she reached back, trying to gather her courage to act. She was a few seconds away from giving it a try when she heard the elevator doors rumble open. A powerful wave of relief instantly swept over her.

"Mom, I'm home," Anise bellowed from the entranceway as she always did.

"In here," she responded in a voice she suspected was too weak to be heard, but before she could call out again, Anise was kneeling at her side.

"What in god's name happened, Mom?" she asked, voice drenched in a mixture of disbelief and panic.

"I fell trying to get to my cell phone."

"Are you okay? How long have you been here like this?"

"Just a couple of minutes. I think I'm okay."

Anise's eyes swelled with tears. She kneeled closer and did the best she could to hug her mom.

"I've got you, Mom. You're going to be okay, but we have to get you back in bed right away."

"Call Dr. Hartzell, honey. Call her right now," Nicole pleaded.

Chapter 9

Being the director of the Division of Elusive Diagnoses at University Hospital in Columbus, Ohio, and a divorced dad left Dr. Jack Wyatt precious little time to spend with his daughter, Anise. Finally, after months of planning and preparation, he was headed east on the Pennsylvania Turnpike toward Washington, DC, to pick her up and embark on a whirlwind college tour. It was the father-daughter trip Jack had been dreaming about since Anise began her freshman year of high school.

The ink had barely dried on their divorce settlement when Nicole's—his now ex-wife—attorney notified Jack that they would be petitioning the court to allow her to move permanently to France with Anise. To support the petition, he cited an outstanding professional opportunity for Nicole and her profound need to be closer to her immediate family. Jack's lawyer strongly objected, but the judge saw things Nicole's way and granted her request. Three months later, Nicole and Anise were unpacking boxes in their Paris apartment overlooking Île Saint-Louis.

Realizing his visitation options were limited, Jack had adjusted to the painful situation by doing everything in his power to travel overseas to visit Anise as often as possible. Other times she would come to Columbus to spend time with him. The arrangement had continued until three years ago when Nicole was aggressively recruited by Marsh Technologies to head up their Global Communications Department. Because it was an incredible opportunity, and she had been toying with the idea of returning to the United States anyway, Nicole had jumped at the chance and accepted the position.

Jack had regrets about the way he'd handled his marriage. He'd been so wrapped up in his practice responsibilities that when the day came that the ax fell and Nicole told him she wanted a divorce, he was still looking the other way. Becoming more introspective about their relationship, he had come to realize he was the one largely responsible for dooming their marriage. He oftentimes wondered whether, if he hadn't been so blithely unaware of her needs, things could have turned out differently.

Jack exited the Pennsylvania Turnpike and headed south on I-71. His navigation system indicated he was two hours and twenty minutes from Nicole's luxury condominium on Connecticut Avenue. He reasoned he had plenty of time to listen to his latest Civil War podcast. About twenty minutes later, he paused the recounting of the Battle of Shiloh and called Anise.

"Hey, Shortstuff. How's my girl?"

"I'm five foot nine, Pops. It may be time for you to come up with a new nickname."

"Not a chance…and actually it was your grandfather who gave you that name."

Jack expected at least a chuckle from his daughter and was surprised by the strained silence that followed his comment.

"I was just about to call you," Anise finally said in a shaky voice.

"You sound upset," he said, hoping their college tour wasn't in jeopardy. "What's going on?"

"Mom's really sick."

"I'm sorry to hear that. You didn't mention anything about it."

"We thought it was just a bad flu and that she'd be better in a few days, but when I came home a little while ago, I found her on the living room floor."

"My god, Anise. Was she conscious?"

"Yes, but I don't think she could have gotten up on her own. She told me she hurt her shoulder. I wanted to call 9-1-1, but she insisted I call her doctor instead."

"And?"

"I spoke with Dr. Hartzell, and she told me to call 9-1-1, but when I told Mom what she said, she refused. She was sure she'd be fine and that she just needed me to help her get back into bed. It took a little while, but we finally managed it. That was about twenty minutes ago. I was just about to call you when you called me."

"And you're sure she's fully conscious and there aren't any bumps or bruises on her head?"

"I'm positive. She told me she didn't hit her head."

"Can she move her arm?"

"Yeah."

"Is she breathing okay?"

"Yes."

"And you think she's okay now?"

"I think so."

Jack's mind pivoted further into its physician mode.

Needing more information, he said, "Start from the beginning and tell me how long Mom's been ill and what her symptoms have been."

"She got sick about five or six days ago, and she won't listen to me or her doctor. You know how she is about her health—she plays everything down and acts like the only thing that can harm her is kryptonite. I…I don't know what to do."

"Has she been getting worse every day?"

"I'd say yes, but she keeps insisting it's just a nasty flu. The one thing that's starting to worry me is that she's been a little confused the past couple of days."

"How confused?"

"She's been forgetful, and sometimes she has trouble following what I'm telling her."

"But her confusion's no worse since the fall?"

"I think it's about the same."

"What did her doctor say when you called her?"

"She said she's not sure what the problem is," Anise answered, falling into the corner of the couch.

"No cough, runny nose, sore throat?"

"No, nothing like that. The first couple of days it was mostly a low-grade fever, a headache, and just feeling weak."

"What's been going on the last two days? Anything different?"

"It's just been more of the same, only worse. She's sleeping more and still has no appetite. Yesterday she told me she was having pins and needles in her fingertips and a lot more trouble moving her arms and legs."

Being a neurologist with a focus on vexing illnesses, Jack didn't like what he was

hearing. His group of potential diagnoses jumped to a short list of worst-case scenarios.

"Did Mom have any idea why she fell?"

"She said she suddenly got dizzy and lost her balance. Like I said, she's been a little confused the last two days, and I don't know how much that had to do with her falling."

"How are you feeling? Are you having any of the same symptoms?"

"Nothing, Pops, I feel absolutely fine."

"What about any of Mom's friends or people she works with? Do you know if any of them were or are ill?"

"I don't know, but Aunt Jenny came over a few days ago for a quick visit. I spoke to her last night and she told me she's fine."

"Has Mom complained about her neck being stiff?"

"No, nothing like that."

Jack reached forward and adjusted the temperature to make his conversion van a few degrees cooler.

"She keeps asking me when you'll be here." A few seconds passed before Anise went on. "Listen, Pops. I know you and Mom have had trouble seeing eye to eye on a lot of things in the past, but she'll never stop believing that you're the world's greatest doctor."

"Tell her I'll be there in about two hours. After I have a chance to have a look at her, we'll figure out what to do next. Now this is the important part—if before I get there you think even for a second that Mom's getting worse, call 9-1-1 immediately. I don't care how much she objects—just call the paramedics… and keep her in bed."

"Okay."

"I'm serious, Shortstuff."

"I've got it. I know what to do."

"Great. What's Mom's doctor's name again?"

"Dr. Kristin Hartzell. She works for Marsh Technologies. She's in charge of the clinic at the corporate headquarters. I checked her out online. I think she's a bigwig at the company. She's been checking in with Mom every day or so."

"I'll let you know when I'm a few minutes away. Everything's going to be fine. Don't worry."

"Pops, Mom and I spend most of our lives worrying about each other. Telling me not to worry about her is like telling a block of ice not to be cold and slippery."

"Call me if anything about Mom's condition changes. Oh, one last thing—besides being a little mixed-up, have you noticed any other changes in her behavior?"

"She been pretty snippy…even for Mom."

Jack couldn't contain a smile. "Anything else?"

"Kind of like I told you; she's been a little confused… and having some trouble with her memory."

"Okay, we'll talk more when I get there. I'll see you in a couple of hours."

The moment Jack ended the call, his sound system returned to the Civil War podcast. Apprehensive about Nicole's illness and wanting to gather his thoughts, he turned it off and switched to an easy-listening channel. Her constellation of symptoms and their severity were sounding an alarm in his head. It was hard for him to draw any firm conclusions from the information Anise had provided him with, but one thing was certain—Nicole wasn't simply battling a severe case of the flu.

Jack couldn't dismiss the possibility that she had contracted an infection of her central nervous system. Although he hadn't disclosed it to Anise, his gut feeling was that she belonged in a hospital where she could get the tests she needed to make a definite diagnosis as quickly as possible. He hoped he'd have a better feel for Nicole's condition after he had the opportunity to see her in person.

Chapter 10

Erik Brickhill was the Marsh Technologies Board of Directors' unanimous choice to serve as the company's fifth CEO. The national search they had conducted seven years earlier had produced a list of impressively qualified candidates. But it was the board's firm opinion that Erik was the only one among them who had the promise of leading the company into the future as one of the country's premier defense contractors. To their delight, he had already skillfully shepherded the company through the process of acquiring several huge defense contracts.

Three days earlier, Erik had responded to Everett Warren's request for an urgent meeting. As it turned out, he'd remember it always as the most vague and unproductive meeting with the board chairman he'd ever attended. It was also the first time he'd found Everett to be an ineffective communicator and visibly nervous and unsure of himself. The only thing Erik learned from the meeting was that Marsh was facing a difficult problem and that he'd be briefed on the details by a consultant in a few days.

Today, as it usually did, his day began at seven a.m. with a breakfast meeting with his executive team. Immediately upon conclusion of the meeting, he chaired the new contracts meeting. It wasn't until ten thirty that he returned to his office. He and had just settled in behind his kidney-shaped mahogany desk when his cell phone rang.

"Erik Brickhill."

Erik suddenly sensed the smart move would be to capitulate to her veiled request. "Assuming I'm able to change my schedule, who'll be attending this meeting?"

"I'm sure you'll find a way to change it—you're the CEO for goodness sakes. And the answer to your question is, just the two of us."

"And what's the agenda to be?" he asked, hoping to get some hint of what was on her mind.

"We'll have plenty of time to talk about the specifics when we meet."

Finally realizing that declining the meeting wasn't an option, he said, "I'll see you at three thirty."

"That's fine. I knew we'd get off to a good start. I look forward to seeing you this afternoon."

"I hope the meeting turns out to be mutually beneficial," he said, feeling a slight headache gathering at the front of his head.

The remainder of Erik's morning was a routine one, spent answering an endless number of emails and phone calls and preparing for the next board of directors meeting. At noon, he informed his assistant he'd decided to go out to lunch. Eating alone was a choice he frequently made. He informed her he'd be back in an hour or so and to please hold his calls unless they were urgent.

Strolling down M Street with the warmth of the sun on his robust shoulders, Erik's mind turned to his impending meeting with Regan Cullen later that afternoon at the Kennedy Center. His plan was simple. As he often did, depending on the nature of the meeting, he'd allow her to do most of the talking until he had an idea of where she was headed.

Chapter 11

To safeguard his custom of eating lunch alone, Erik tended to choose from a select few restaurants that were within walking distance of the corporate headquarters. On this particular day, he chose one that offered Peruvian food in a casual dining environment. He was well acquainted with the owner, who always held a table for him in a stone alcove at the back of the restaurant.

He was perusing the menu when a smartly dressed woman approached his table. He raised his eyes and smiled at her politely before turning his attention back to the menu. When she pulled out the chair across from him and sat down, he was naturally surprised, but he guarded his silence. Even though he'd only spoken to her briefly on the phone, he had an inkling of who his uninvited lunch guest was.

"You don't look surprised," she said to him with a chuckle, slinging her purse over the back of the chair. "I guess your reputation for being unflappable is well deserved. I'm Regan."

"Aren't you a little early and in the wrong place for our meeting?"

"I was feeling a little guilty about disturbing your afternoon schedule, so I decided to move things up."

"But not guilty enough to give me a call and let me know about it."

"I thought it would be better this way." She didn't have to spell it out for him. Obviously, she didn't trust him and wanted to be assured their meeting would be absolutely private.

"Would you like to see a menu?" Erik asked.

"Heavens no. I generally skip lunch, but you go ahead and order. I probably won't be here that long. I just wanted to meet you in person because, as your consultant, I think it's essential to keep the lines of communication open between us, especially when facing a crisis of this magnitude."

"Since I don't know what the exact nature of the crisis is, it would be hard for me to comment on that."

"That's the good part for you—it's not essential that you know the details." She glanced around and then leaned her head over the table. "You should feel free to call me Regan. I prefer first names. We're going to be facing some tough problems in the next couple of weeks. The reason I'm here is to make sure that, moving forward, we're on the same page. I'm not a back-of-the-boat-type person staring at where we've been. I prefer the front. That way I can concentrate on where we're headed."

"Consultant?" he asked her. "I'm going to make an assumption. This crisis you're referring to took place on U.S. soil, which would mean you're not CIA."

"To my way of thinking, Washington's got so many offices, bureaus, and agencies that they're all just one big alphabet soup. I like to think of all of us as one big crew team with everybody rowing in the same direction." Tossing in a mild shrug, she added, "Names—and especially acronyms—don't mean anything. Don't you agree?"

He cringed inwardly at her hokey, overly dramatic style of communication. It was entirely too pretentious and put-on for his taste.

"That's an interesting way of looking at it." He was trying his best not to sound skeptical or make her think he wasn't taking her seriously.

She reached into her white Library of Congress canvas tote bag, pulled out a roll of Life Savers, and popped one in her mouth.

"Do you have any questions for me regarding the operation?"

"I wasn't aware there was an operation. Is it already under way?"

"Yes."

"From what little Everett Warren told me, I suspect it involves our employees. I'd like to know how many."

"I'm sorry, I can't tell you that."

"I see," he said, holding up a hand to signal the approaching server he wasn't ready.

"I can sense your frustration, so let me simplify things for you. All I need from you is to answer any questions that I might have in the next week or so. If you leave the nuts and bolts of the operation to me, I promise you, everything will be just fine."

"That's good to hear," he said apathetically.

A brief but strained silence ensued.

"On second thought, perhaps, it would be a good idea for me to clarify a couple of things for you. Anything that happened in the past is irrelevant. We're just going to have to deal with the collateral damage. But you should know that we're really up against the clock on this thing. It's my job to make certain the situation is handled expeditiously and permanently."

He pushed his palms together as he spoke. "I'm getting the feeling from you and Everett that, whatever this crisis is, it's creating an accelerated hysteria."

"What's your point?"

"Is it remotely possible the parties involved are seriously over-reacting?"

"No, it's not possible," Regan said flatly. "Marsh Technologies is counted among the elite of our country's defense contractors. We're not looking for your approval. The strategic decisions that have been made are so far above your pay grade you'd need the Hubble tele-scope to see them. Our marching orders come from the top and it's my job to help in sparing the federal government any embarrass-ment or harm." She pressed her hands flat on the table with a look on her face and an inflection in her voice that were no longer light-hearted. "Your country needs you to be a loyal American. Tell me you've got it, Erik—and tell me we won't have to have this conversation again."

He responded with a simple nod.

"I'd prefer a yes or no response."

Erik was a man of discipline and restraint, but he had just so much patience for uncivil people who might confuse his courtesy for weakness. Normally, he might elevate the intensity of the conversation, based on the way Regan had just taken him to the woodshed, but something instinctual prompted him not to act on the impulse.

"Yes, I've got it, and no, it won't be necessary to have this conversation again. Was there something else you wanted to speak to me about?"

"I do have a question," she said. "Do you have concerns that anybody on your executive staff might know something that they wouldn't be comfortable sharing with you?"

"I don't think so. But since I'm not a mind reader, I can't be entirely positive."

"Good, and thanks for the straight answer. I prefer things that way. It's my expectation that in a matter of days things could become very challenging from a public relations standpoint. What's your level of confidence in your public relations department?"

"I think they do a good job. If you'll provide me with sufficient guidance, our executive team will be able to brief them on all public statements and responses to the media's questions."

"Excellent. And of course the appropriate information and guidelines will be provided to you," she said, reaching for her tote bag. "The next week or so will be critical. You'll almost certainly become aware of things that seem odd or confusing. Don't overreact to them. It's important to keep your wits about you." She pushed her chair back and stood up. Erik didn't follow, nor did he say anything. "I'll probably be reaching out to you again in a day or so to set up another meeting."

"I'll expect your call."

"Oh, there's one last thing. You might want to think about

checking your attitude at the door and just try to take things in stride. You're a pretty bright guy, but I assure you, you're not the smartest person in the room...and you're not a Supreme Court justice."

"Translate," he said plainly, observing the tenacity in her eyes.

"Your position at Marsh isn't a lifetime appointment. Don't let some pious attack of conscience prompt you to do something dumb. Watch your six, Erik. This isn't your Thursday-night poker game with your ex-Marine Corps buddies where the worst thing that can happen is you lose a few bucks." Without waiting for a response, she turned and headed toward the exit.

"Thank you for the advice," he muttered to himself as he signaled the server.

While he waited for his lunch, he reflected on his meeting with Regan. He suspected Everett wouldn't be overjoyed with his level of enthusiasm, but he'd done nothing to blatantly disregard his instructions. Erik was capable of bending over backward to be a team player—but not to a point where his spine would crack. He detested the thought of being an effusive ass-kisser, but not having the details of the crisis made it near impossible for him to decide upon the best way to conduct himself moving forward.

Chapter 12

An hour and fifty minutes after his conversation with Anise, Jack pulled up to Nicole's stately pre-war construction building. The valet, an eager young man wearing a snug red vest, jogged up to his van.

"We don't see a lot of conversion vans like this. You must be Dr. Wyatt."

"I am," he said, maneuvering his athletic frame out of the van. "You've obviously spoken to my daughter."

"She called me about an hour ago. My name's Eddie. I'll be taking care of your vehicle for you. Just check in at the welcome desk. They're expecting you." Jack reached into his pocket, but Eddie grinned politely. "We have a no-tipping policy, Doc." Jack smiled right back at him and left the five-dollar bill on the front seat.

"When I was in high school, I spent my summers as a busboy. The experience left me strongly opposed to no-tipping policies." Eddie chuckled but said nothing.

Jack entered the lobby through a revolving glass door, registered at the security desk, and rode the elevator to the seventh floor. When the doors rolled open, Anise was there to meet him. Her lips were quivering, and the soft tissues beneath her eyes were puffy from sobbing. As she hugged her dad, she could barely hold back a new flood of tears.

"I'm so glad you're here, Pops."

"We're going to sort this out, and everything's going to be okay. How's Mom been since we spoke—any changes?"

"She's about the same."

"C'mon, let's go see her."

Anise escorted him through the spacious living room with its lavish modernistic styling. Jack caught a glimpse of the Potomac River and the Washington Monument through the double-glazed glass wall before they made their way down the main hallway to the master suite.

The door was open, and they quietly stepped into Nicole's room. The clammy scent of illness was in the air. Nicole was dimly visible in the bed until Anise opened the curtains. The moment Jack set eyes on her, his worst fears were realized. Whatever hope he had that she might not need to be hospitalized vanished faster than a spark of electricity. Her face was the color of chalk, her breathing was a little irregular, and her lips were framed by patches of flaky skin.

At first, she didn't realize Jack and Anise were in the room. Just as he was about to say something, she shifted her gaze to him.

"Hi, Jack. I'm so glad you're here." Her face was wrinkled with distress. "It's been a tough week."

"Anise filled me in on what's been going on and what happened earlier today."

"She worries about me way too much."

"I think that's something you both do when it comes to each other. How's your shoulder?"

"It's feeling much better. I think I just bruised it a little."

He walked to the bedside. While he gently examined her shoulder, he asked, "Compared to when all this started, have you been feeling any better in the last day or two?"

"Not really, but I've had worse days."

"Really? When was that?"

"I'd have to think about it," she answered, averting her eyes ever so slightly, a harmless

tendency of hers Jack had long ago noted when she was caught not being totally forthcoming.

"Listen, Nicole. I understand you're pretty stoic when it comes to your health, but I need you to be honest with me about how you're feeling."

"If you insist. I feel like a large drawbridge collapsed on me."

"Anise told me you've been sick for about a week. What were the very first symptoms you noticed?" he asked as he examined her neck. It was supple, and she had no pain when he gently flexed it.

"It was mostly just a bad headache and being exhausted."

"Fever?"

"I don't think so, but I can't be sure…maybe a little," she answered in a voice that wobbled. She reached for a glass of water that was sitting on her nightstand. Jack noticed her motion was uncoordinated, and her hand was trembling. Anise flew to the bedside, picked up the glass before Nicole could, and helped her place the tip of the straw between her lips.

When she was finished drinking, Jack asked, "And what happened over the next few days and up until now?"

"I don't know. It's hard to remember. The days are kind of flowing together." Jack decided to make his questions more targeted to help Nicole formulate an answer.

"Have you noticed any numbness in your hands or feet?"

"My fingers have been tingling for a few days."

"Dizziness?"

"Some, I guess, but it's the headache and this brain fog that are really bothering me."

"Where's the headache?"

"In the front, and it hasn't moved."

"Does it come and go or make you sick to your stomach?"

"No. It's there all the time.

"What about the weakness in your arms and legs? Is it better or worse?"

"I'd say a little worse."

"Anise said you haven't done any traveling lately."

"She hasn't, Pops."

"What about recent vaccinations? Have you had any?"

"No…I don't think so."

"Have you noticed any insect bites or been around anybody who's been ill?"

She waved her hand side to side. "No."

Jack was becoming more concerned about her breathing with each question he asked. Her sentences were chopped, and her efforts to speak were leaving her more breathless with each word she uttered. Increasingly more concerned that Nicole's oxygen reserves could be approaching low levels, he decided not to stress her any further with more questions. His mind shifted to the most pressing issue, which was to get Nicole transported to a hospital as quickly as possible.

"What the hell's wrong with me, Jack?"

"That's what we're going to figure out, but your condominium isn't the place to do that."

"If you take me to the ER, they'll just send me home with some Tylenol."

"I'm not talking about a visit to the emergency room. You need to be admitted."

She waved a hand in objection. "Jack, I really don't—"

"C'mon, Mom. You have to do what Dad says. There's no reason to say no. I'm calling Dr. Hartzell and we're taking you to the hospital."

"It's for the best, Nicole. And please don't try to speak any more. It's making it harder for you to breathe."

The room went silent, and Jack could see the capitulation in her eyes. He knew, whether she agreed with him or not, she didn't have the mental or physical strength to resist any longer.

Jack had always been a believer that first impressions were important. It was a belief he relied on when it came to making a difficult diagnosis. Even though he had relatively little to go on, his mind was already rifling through the possibilities as to what might be causing Nicole's illness. The combination and severity of her symptoms plus their steady progression left him well beyond worried. The next most logical step was to speak with Dr. Hartzell to see what she could add to further his understanding of Nicole's illness. He glanced at Anise, who covertly pointed toward the door.

"Excuse us for a second, Nicole," he said in a voice punctuated with calmness.

"We'll be right back, Mom," Anise said, following Jack out into the hall and then into the living room.

What's wrong with Mom, Pops? And please tell me the truth."

"I think she may have encephalitis. It's an infection of the brain."

"Like meningitis?"

"Meningitis affects the lining of the brain and spinal cord, but the two can be present at the same time. I can't be certain, but I don't think Mom has meningitis."

She stared at him in disbelief. Her eyes pooled with tears.

"How in the world would she get an infection of her brain?"

"There are a few ways, but we can talk about that later. Right now, while I'm calling 9-1-1, I want you to contact the security desk and see if they keep emergency oxygen in the building. If they do, tell them we need it right away. When you're finished, see if you can get Dr. Hartzell on the phone. I'd like to speak with her."

"I'm so scared, Pops. I don't know if I can…"

"Sure you can. Take a breath, stay focused, and make the calls."

Jack reached for his phone, called 9-1-1, and gave the dispatcher the information she required to send an ambulance.

"No oxygen," Anise said, hurrying back into the living room. "I left a message for Dr. Hartzell."

"Good."

"How long before the paramedics get here?" she asked.

"Assuming they're on their way. It shouldn't be too long."

"Mom's going to be okay…right, Pops?"

"If I have anything to say about it, she will. C'mon, let's go back to her room."

Jack helped Nicole sit up a little higher. "The ambulance is on the way, and we've notified Dr. Hartzell."

Her only response was a weak attempt at a smile and a frail wave of capitulation. He continued to study her face for any clues of an impending crisis. Observing she was having difficulty focusing, he checked his watch again. It had been seven minutes since he'd called for assistance. Jack was acutely aware of one reality—the sooner Nicole got to a hospital, the better. Her neurologic symptoms were advanced, and he was concerned she could suffer a seizure at any time.

Anise's cell phone rang. She checked the caller ID. "It's Dr. Hartzell," she said as she walked to the other side of the room.

She answered the call and took a minute to explain what had happened. She listened for a minute or so, slowly nodding her head. "Thank you, Dr. Hartzell. I'll let my dad know."

Jack walked over and joined her. "What did she say?"

"She's going to make sure the paramedics transport Mom to Georgetown Infirmary and bring her straight to the ICU on the fourth floor. She wants us to wait for her there. She said she'll be out to talk with you as soon as she's sure Mom's stable." Before Jack could respond, Anise's phone rang again. "Thanks, Mike," she said as she gave her dad a thumbs-up. "That was the desk. The ambulance just pulled up in front of the building. Mike's going to bring the paramedics straight up."

"Why don't you go meet them at the elevator. I'll stay here with Mom."

It didn't take long for the two paramedics to enter the apartment and make their way back to the master suite. Jack identified himself as a physician and briefed them on the urgency of Nicole's condition. While he was doing so, the two young women worked quickly to start her on high-flow oxygen, get a set of vital signs, and insert an IV in her left forearm. They were obviously experienced and understood those times in medicine when efficiency together with speed can make an important difference in patient outcome.

They loaded Nicole onto the stretcher. Once she was securely in place, they confirmed with Jack that Dispatch had informed them to transport her to Georgetown Infirmary. With Jack and Anise right behind them, they wheeled the stretcher back to the elevator, down to the lobby, and out to the ambulance. After a brief period of time to get her secured, they made a radio transmission and sped off with lights and sirens.

Chapter 13

With its multicolored strobes flashing, the ambulance carrying Nicole Wyatt backed into the receiving bay of the Georgetown Infirmary's emergency room. In its brief seven-year history, the two-hundred-bed hospital had developed the reputation of serving DC's most notable carriage trade. Since its inception, its mission had been to deliver world-class care while providing a concierge-level patient experience. Helping them to realize their mission was a financial bedrock as solid as any hospital in the country.

Marsh Technologies believed in a progressive healthcare program for their employees. Five years earlier they had established a relationship with the Infirmary where they would be the principal facility responsible for caring for any Marsh employee who required admission to a hospital.

Jack and Anise arrived fifteen minutes after the ambulance. The white-haired gentleman staffing the lobby's welcome center provided them each with a visitor's pass and directed them to the unit on the fourth floor. They stepped off the elevator and followed a short corridor lined with outdoor marketplace watercolors that led them to the entrance of the critical care units. They entered and were a few feet from the core desk when a young nurse in royal blue scrubs and an engaging smile greeted them.

"May I help you?"

"I'm Jack Wyatt. This is my daughter Anise. We're—"

She extended her hand. "It's very nice to meet you both. My name's Melony. I'm the assistant nurse manager of the unit. Dr. Hartzell told me to expect you."

"Is my mom okay?" Anise was quick to ask with breathless anticipation.

"Dr. Hartzell and her team are in with her now. I just checked a minute ago, and I was told she's responding well to treatment." She turned to Jack. "If you and Anise will have a seat in the waiting room, I'll let Dr. Hartzell know you're here. She wanted me to let you know she'll be out to speak with you as soon as she's able. If you need anything, there's a phone in the waiting room that's a direct line to the nursing station."

"Thank you," Jack said, seeing no reason to pose any additional questions, especially in the presence of Anise. Melony turned and headed back down the hall toward Nicole's room.

"Try to stay calm. We'll know more after we speak to Dr. Hartzell," he assured her, gesturing toward the exit. Anise walked alongside him as they headed toward the waiting room. "These types of illnesses are tough to figure. A lot of people recover from them almost as fast as they got them."

"Please, Pops. I know Mom's really sick," she said, her voice resonating with fear.

"You have to remember that Mom knows what you're thinking almost before you do. Do your best to stay optimistic when you see her."

"I'll give it my best shot, but you're the one who's always telling me I wear my emotions on my sleeve."

Once they entered the waiting room, Anise pointed toward the back where they sat down on a beige love seat. Twenty minutes later, a woman wearing a knee-length navy-blue lab coat and walking at a brisk pace approached them.

"You must be Dr. Wyatt. My name's Kristin Hartzell. Although

I wish it were under different circumstances, it's a pleasure to meet you." Turning to Anise, she added, "It's nice to finally meet you in person as well."

Kristin had been accepted to each of the nine top-tier U.S. medical schools she'd applied to but had decided to study medicine in Dublin at the Royal College of Surgeons. After being awarded her medical degree, she was accepted as a resident in internal medicine at Georgetown University School of Medicine where, upon completion of her training, she stayed on as a junior faculty member. But after eleven years of too many mind-bending eighteen-hour days and nights on call, she finally came to grips with her emotional exhaustion and decided her personal and professional survival depended on her making a change.

When she was approached by a recruiter from Marsh Technologies to consider a newly created position as their first chief visionary medical officer, she found the prospect intriguing. After the team at Marsh courted her like a rock star, she overlooked the doubts she still harbored and decided that this was one of those times in life when you just had to hold your nose and jump. That was five years ago, and as it turned out, she'd never looked back. She found exploring new and innovative initiatives in healthcare delivery both challenging and exciting. At the same time, she was able to keep her hand in clinical medicine by heading up a medical wellness center at Marsh's corporate headquarters.

She took Anise's hands in hers. "The paramedics did a great job stabilizing your mom, but I won't kid you, she's pretty sick. Right now, she's holding her own. We started her on several medications, including a strong antibiotic. We're also in the process of doing a lot of blood tests and some x-rays. We've given her a hefty dose of sedation, and for now she's resting comfortably." She spoke with a flat calm in her voice.

"Do you know what's making her so sick?"

"We have some ideas, but we won't be positive about anything until we get the results of our tests back."

"How long will that take?"

"I wish I could answer that question, but it's hard to know when the various labs will finish the tests and send us the results."

With a distraught face, Anise regarded each of them in turn. "Would it be okay if I sat with her for a little while? I'd like to be there with her when she wakes up."

"Of course. She's in room 4006. Melony will escort you. In the meantime, I'll fill your dad in on some of the medical details. It'll be a lot of doctor talk, but if your dad says it's okay, you're welcome to stay and listen."

"Thank you, but I think I should be with my mom."

Jack took a few steps forward and gave Anise a quick hug.

"I'll meet you in Mom's room as soon as Dr. Hartzell and I are finished talking."

"Okay."

Watching Anise make her way toward the entrance to the critical care units took a heavy emotional toll on him. Even though he'd been separated from Anise geographically for several years, they had managed to maintain a close relationship where Jack always felt sure they could discuss and work out any problem she faced. He now found himself wondering if events in the days to come might shake his confidence in that belief.

He knew Anise expected him to find a way to make sure Nicole would fully recover and restore her life to normal. She had always viewed him as a superhero who could fix anything. He dreaded the thought of failing her, but the doctor in him knew that not all cases of encephalitis were curable, and what the future held for Nicole might be the worst-case scenario. Jack knew his first priority was to stay focused, which meant doing everything in his power to remain objective and park his emotional side in some remote corner of his mind.

He was suddenly snapped back to the here and now by the sound of Kristin's voice.

"There's a physician's library just down the hall. I suggest we speak there. It'll give us a little more privacy."

"That sounds fine," he said, anxious to get Kristin's take on Nicole's illness.

Chapter 14

While they walked down the corridor toward the library, Jack and Kristin's conversation remained casual, neither of them broaching the topic of Nicole's illness. Opening the door, she waited for Jack to enter. The library was of moderate size and smartly appointed. The finely crafted dark-wood bookshelves housed a mixture of medical textbooks and journals. The carpet was a plush gray. In the center of the room sat a boat-shaped conference table.

"Please have a seat," she said, pointing to one of the six leather chairs that were arranged around the table. "Nicole told me a couple of days ago that you'd be arriving today. She also mentioned that you're a neurologist. I imagine you're already aware that she was quite insistent that I brief you on her condition."

"Both Nicole and Anise mentioned it to me."

"I get the feeling they both hold you in pretty high esteem."

"That's kind of you to say," Jack responded, before adding, "I was interested to learn you work exclusively for Marsh."

"I do, but it seems like every time I mention it to a colleague, they look at me as if I've sold my soul to the medical devil."

Jack chuckled. "Believe me, I have no preconceived notions about what it's like to work for a large private corporation, Dr.

Hartzell. But I do work for a big university with their own set of strange ideas as to how best to provide healthcare. I'd bet there are more similarities than differences between our respective situations."

"You're probably right, and please call me Kristin." The relaxed look fell from her face, pushed aside by a more solemn one. "Before I brief you on Nicole's condition, do you have any questions for me?"

"I don't think so. I'd prefer to hear your impressions of her illness first…if that's okay with you."

"That's fine," Kristin said, sitting back in her chair and turning it just slightly to the side. "The first time I saw Nicole was in our wellness center at Marsh's corporate headquarters. She'd been sick for about a day and a half. She didn't strike me as particularly ill. My impression was she'd contracted a viral illness that would run its course and resolve on its own in a few days. I didn't order any lab tests or x-rays or prescribe any medications," she explained, her voice confident. "When I saw her back in the clinic two days later, she was clearly worse. Her principal complaints were a persistent headache and a generalized weakness. I felt her examination was normal, and although my level of concern was higher, I still felt she was suffering from a self-limited viral illness. I didn't think she needed to be admitted to our hospital, but I did order routine blood work that included a standard viral panel. I had the results a couple of hours later, and everything was basically normal."

"I assume the viral panel included a flu and Covid assay, and that it was negative."

She nodded and said, "I told her to stay home and that I'd check on her by phone the following day. When I spoke to her then, I thought she was about the same, but when I talked to her yesterday, I was definitely more concerned. Her neurologic symptoms had worsened, which prompted me to strongly suggest she come here to the ER, where I would meet her. I told her that, based on my assessment in the emergency department, I might recommend she be admitted to the hospital."

"Knowing how Nicole feels about hospitals, I'm not surprised she rejected your advice."

"She did promise to call me back and meet me in the ER if she started to feel worse," Kristin was quick to respond, rapidly tapping her fingertips together. "I was just getting ready to check on her today when I received Anise's call that you had arrived and were making arrangements for her to be urgently transported." With a face bathed in apprehension, Kristin stood up, walked behind her chair and curled her fingers around the top. From her manner and voice, he got the impression there was something more alarming on her mind. "Nicole suffered a seizure while the paramedics were bringing her up to the unit. It continued for a few minutes, but we were able to get it under control. I think we're okay for now, but I don't have the first clue what the next few hours might bring."

Jack was disquieted, but not stunned, to hear the news. The possibility of a seizure had been his major fear from the moment he'd laid eyes on Nicole. Its occurrence made him more convinced than ever she was suffering from encephalitis.

"Did you have to put her on a ventilator?"

"No, but I'd say it's a real possibility, especially if the seizures recur."

"It's been my experience in this setting that they oftentimes do."

"Unfortunately, Nicole has another finding that's equally concerning," Kristin said. "We fear she may have an impending lower extremity paralysis. There's no history of a tick or mosquito bite, but my working diagnosis is viral encephalitis." She held her next thought long enough to retake her seat. "Would you agree?"

"I'd agree that encephalitis would be at the top of my short list of diagnostic possibilities." Being a neurologist and having cared for numerous patients suffering from the disease, Jack had an extensive amount of experience diagnosing and treating it. The types of viral encephalitis that spread from person to person varied considerably in how contagious they were. Sophisticated tests were now available that could specifically identify the particular strain of virus, but there were many cases, some that ended in death, where the offending virus was never discovered. The seizure was a disheartening development and almost certainly foretold that Nicole's road to recovery would be an arduous one. "Do you have any of the test results back yet?"

"Just a few and so far they've been pretty much normal. I'm waiting for the spinal tap results. We have her scheduled for an MRI in an hour. Obviously, that's assuming she's stable for transport to the MRI suite. I've also sent off an extensive panel of viral studies, including PCR testing from her blood and spinal fluid. She hasn't had any recent vaccines or recurrent illnesses from the past, so I think we can assume an autoimmune encephalitis isn't likely." She paused briefly. Jack could see the trepidation in her eyes. Finally, she asked plainly, "Is there anything else you can think of?"

"In my opinion, your diagnostic workup has been comprehensive and complete. Until the test results start coming back, I'd say the only sensible option you have is supportive care. If encephalitis does turn out to be the diagnosis, hopefully the lab will be able to isolate the specific virus that's causing it."

Kristin responded cautiously, "Which will only mean something if we have a currently available antiviral drug that turns out to be effective against it." Jack waited, expecting her to expand on her thoughts, but to his surprise, she didn't. With her forehead bunched together, she finally stated, "I don't think the problem's as straightforward as it appears. Earlier today, I admitted a thirty-two-year-old woman, also a Marsh employee, who just happens to work on the same floor as Nicole. She's also been ill for the past week with symptoms that, for all intents and purposes, are identical to Nicole's."

Jack was more than a little taken aback by Kristin's disclosure. He agreed with her that it might be a significant piece of information.

"It could turn out later not to be important," he said. "But I wouldn't dismiss any possibility out of hand this early into your diagnostic evaluation."

"My understanding is that viral encephalitis is usually caused by a tick or a mosquito bite and is a pretty uncommon disease. It's also not very contagious."

"That's usually the case, but there are exceptions," Jack said. "Overall, herpes simplex is the most common virus that causes encephalitis. Generally, tick and mosquito bites occur at certain times of the year where those insects are endemic. In Nicole's case, eastern equine encephalitis would be the most likely diagnosis. It's also worth mentioning that the vast majority of cases occur in the Gulf and Eastern states from July to September."

Crossing her fingers and holding them up, she said, "It's November, so that's at least one break in our favor." For the first time, Jack sensed her words were choked with apprehension.

"Have you seen any other cases in your clinic with symptoms similar to Nicole's?"

"A number of patients this week came in with flu-like symptoms, but that's not uncommon for this time of the year. Your question is an excellent one. I'm afraid I can't dismiss the possibility there could be other cases lagging behind Nicole's.

"If there are more cases, could they be in other hospitals?" Jack asked.

"It's possible but not likely. I generally find out about any Marsh patients in other emergency rooms who require admission. As soon as I do, we make arrangements to have them transferred here to the Infirmary."

"In that case, there's not much you can do other than sit tight and see what happens over the next few days." Taking the conversation in a different direction, he asked, "What's your feeling about starting Nicole and your other patient on an antiviral drug, even though you don't have a positive test for a specific virus?"

"Actually, I ordered them both started on ganciclovir. After we get the results of their PCRs, spinal fluid analyses, and cultures, we can make whatever drug change we need to."

"I agree."

"Any other thoughts or suggestions?" she asked him.

"It sounds to me like you've done everything by the book. All you can do at this point is provide supportive care and be ready to act on any new test results that indicate a change in therapy."

"Thanks, Jack…and if moving forward you have any other ideas on the diagnosis or treatment, I'd greatly appreciate it if you'd share them with me."

"Of course," Jack said, starting to wonder if Kristin knew a little bit more about his specialized practice than she was letting on.

"In that case, I know you must be anxious to join Anise, and I should get back to Nicole."

"Thanks for taking the time to speak with me."

They stood up and headed toward the door.

APPROACHING the entrance to the unit, Jack again found himself wondering if Georgetown Infirmary had seen its last case of encephalitis. He realized it would be pure speculation to assume there would be more. In a way, it wasn't of great importance at the moment. His feeling was that Kristin's approach had to focus on the two patients she was currently treating. From a pragmatic stand-point, if more Marsh employees with encephalitis presented to the Infirmary, she'd just have to find a way to deal with the problem.

Chapter 15

Jack was still pondering his conversation with Kristin when he walked through the door of Nicole's room. Finding both her and Anise asleep, he quietly made his way over to the bedside.

Nicole's breathing was slightly more labored, and her face had the same sallow complexion. He glanced at the multicolored monitor displays over her bed. Her pulse, blood pressure, and the amount of oxygen she was carrying in her blood were all in acceptable ranges, but he remained worried Nicole still hadn't seen the worst of the illness.

For reasons that exceeded his understanding, Jack had a nagging feeling that Marsh Technologies' two cases of encephalitis were not going to be straightforward. Even with his extensive experience as a neurologist, including his special expertise in the diagnosis of elusive illnesses, a strange feeling chewed at his gut that there was something more complex about the disease than met the eye and that determining the cause would be a challenge.

Jack moved to the other side of the room and gently tapped Anise on her shoulder. Her eyes snapped open.

"Mom's doing okay for the moment. Why don't I take you back to the condo?"

She quietly lowered the footrest of the lounger and came to her feet.

"I think I should stay until she wakes up."

"Dr. Hartzell has her heavily sedated. She's going to sleep for hours. You'll be able to come back later to see her."

Anise walked over to the bed. Looking at her mother through tear-laden eyes, she slowly leaned over and kissed her cheek. She then gently pushed a few stubborn strands of Nicole's reddish-brown hair from her forehead. Nicole didn't stir a bit.

"Okay, Pops."

They exited the hospital into a windy afternoon with low-lying stacks of ominous looking clouds obscuring the sun's light.

Jack gestured across the street to a large sandwich shop with a red awning.

"What do you say we grab something to eat before heading back to the condo?"

They quick-stepped across the street and entered the restaurant, where they were seated and handed two menus. A couple of minutes passed before an overworked appearing server walked over to the table.

"Are you ready to order?" he asked impatiently, tilting his head back and forth like a metronome.

"I think we are," Jack said.

"Shoot."

"I'll have a ham and gouda melt, and the young lady will have a Greek salad."

"To drink?

"Two waters with lemon, please."

"You got it," he said, tapping his bottom lip with the eraser end of his pencil.

As soon as he stepped away, Anise said, "I'm sorry about our college tour, Pops."

"The importance of the trip pales in comparison to your mom's illness…and you said that as if any of this is your fault."

"I should have called you sooner."

"First of all that's not true and secondly, let's not dwell on what's passed. The only thing that matters now is getting her better. I assure you, we'll have plenty of time to make the trip when Mom's fully recovered." Moving to another topic, he asked, "How's the application process going?"

"I'm worried that too many of the schools we picked are stretches. We need at least one more safe school. I'm starting to feel like I'll be lucky to get in anywhere."

Jack didn't respond at first. He unwrapped his napkin and removed the silverware.

"Let's see. You're a National Merit Scholar who's sure to graduate in the top five percent of her class. You probably have more extracurricular activities than any other high school student on the East Coast, and you're the captain of both the lacrosse and forensics team… Oh yeah, and let's not forget that you killed the SAT and that you speak French fluently." He paused and opened his hands with his palms turned upward. "Yeah, you're probably right. With such a mediocre high school record of achievement, what college admissions committee would possibly be interested in offering you a spot in their freshman class?"

She gave it her best shot to hold a straight face, but the corners of her mouth turned up into an amused smile.

"I hope you're right," was all she could manage. "Since you're obviously not going to tell me unless I ask—what did Dr. Hartzell say was making Mom so sick?"

"It's still too early to say, since there are a bunch of test results pending and others to be scheduled. It's mostly a waiting game at this point. The results of the tests are going to be key."

"When will we know?"

"It's going to vary, but as Dr. Hartzell said, it should be over the next few days."

"But you both think she has encephalitis?"

"Nothing's for sure but that's what we're leaning toward."

"I've already checked the internet. It sounds like a horrible disease. I don't really think she was bitten by a tick, Pops, so how in the world did she get it?"

"There are several different types of encephalitis and several different ways of getting it. We're going to need some more time to figure all that out."

"Is it contagious…I mean, did she catch it from somebody else?"

"It's remotely possible but not likely. Some people who get viral encephalitis are pretty sick, just like Mom, but the vast majority of them have no symptoms or mild ones. Even once the virus is in somebody's body, it's rare for it to cause encephalitis." Jack had a pretty good idea where Anise was taking him with her questions. He was surprised at first when she didn't ask him directly if there was a chance Nicole might die. He had no doubt the possibility had crossed her mind, but he suspected she hadn't summoned the courage yet to talk about it.

"Are you going to be involved in Mom's care…I mean officially?"

"Dr. Hartzell hasn't brought up the possibility."

"If she does ask you, would it include Madison?"

"I don't know, but I'm going to discuss everything that's happened so far when I pick her up at the airport tonight. Do you want to come with me?"

"I'd like to, but Aunt Jenny's really worried about Mom and wants me to come over and fill her in on things. I'll probably head back to the hospital after leaving her house."

"That sounds fine. I'll give her a call later."

"How's Madison feeling? I should have asked sooner. I'm sorry. I can almost hear Mom telling me not to forget my manners."

Jack tapped the tabletop twice with his knuckles for good luck.

"Madison's doing fine. She sees her hematologist regularly, and all the reports have been great." He added, "You're being a little tough on yourself about not asking. You're going through your own crisis right now, and nobody would understand that better than Madison."

"How long after somebody's in remission from leukemia until they're considered cured?"

"I guess that can vary quite a bit depending on the type of leukemia, especially with all the genetic studies they're doing these days. Although she's doing great, I don't think her doctors feel she's out of the woods yet. If you'd like to, I'm sure she wouldn't mind talking to you about it."

"Maybe I'll wait for the right moment and bring it up."

Jack hesitated briefly before asking, "Have you spoken to her about us getting married and her being your..."

"My stepmom? Not yet, Pops."

"How come?"

"It's a little hard to explain."

"Try me."

"We don't exactly have that kind of relationship. Sometimes, I kind of get the feeling she thinks I'm her number one competitor for you."

"I never realized you felt that way. She's never said anything to me that would make me even the slightest bit suspicious she feels that way."

"It's a girl thing, and don't get me wrong—I like Madison a lot, and I have tons of admiration for her. We get along fine. We're just not that close...yet." She looked up at Jack, shook her head, and said, "And, Pops, I seriously doubt she'd mention anything to you about this one little bump in our relationship."

"I'll tell you what, let's put this topic on the back burner for now. It's important, and I'm not saying we abandon it, but for right now you need to feel comfortable focusing all your attention on Mom."

"Okay, but I promise, as soon as Mom's better, I'll take Madison out to lunch, and I'll do everything I can to get our friendship to the next level."

"Sounds like a plan," he said, realizing she was getting older and was able to handle these types of little challenges without too much of his input.

Anise hadn't really told him anything he wasn't already aware of. He didn't think there was a problem between them, but he also realized there was room for improvement. Seeing as how they were both warm and emotionally mature people, he assumed once they opened the lines of communication, things would work out fine.

While they ate their lunch, Jack fielded several more medical questions. He was for the most part forthcoming, but at times he intentionally responded vaguely or sidestepped Anise's questions the best he could. He did, however, make it clear that her mom's road to recovery might be a long and rocky one. Just as importantly, he assured her he'd make himself available to Dr. Hartzell whenever she wished to speak with him.

It wasn't hard for him to see that Anise was hanging on to his every word and doing her best to remain composed. Jack knew how dearly she loved Nicole. She was her best friend and hero. It was no surprise that the thought of losing her left her feeling like she was hanging on to the lowest rung of the ladder.

Chapter 16

For the past six days, John Winkler had been battling the worst case of the flu he could remember in decades. It was an unusually warm day for November, prompting him to slowly make his way to their patio room where he found a seat in his favorite lounger. Trying to take his mind off his illness, he looked out over the vast wooded area behind the house. He tried to focus his eyes to counteract the double vision he'd been suffering since earlier that morning, but he was only partially successful.

After a few labored breaths, he reached down, mustered all the strength he could, and yanked on the wooden handle that elevated the footrest. Picking up his wool blanket, he opened it the best he could and then draped it across his bony legs and abdomen. Having missed four days of work at Marsh, he was tempted to call their clinic, but after some further thought, he decided to give it another day, hoping he'd start to feel better.

Massaging the sides of his head did little to diminish the headache that had been throbbing incessantly for the past four days. The weakness in his arms and hands that he'd first noticed two days ago had also worsened overnight. Just then, his wife, Annette, strolled into the room with a mug of piping hot green tea. She was three years older than he, had her masters in speech pathology, and was one of the few people on earth who could manage John's many moods.

"Feeling any better?" she asked, setting the mug down on the small glass table next to the lounger.

"Not yet," he answered, rolling his fingertips together, trying to get some relief from the maddening pins and needles that were getting worse with each passing hour.

"YOUR STUBBORNNESS IS SHOWING, honey. Maybe it's time you went to the ER or saw Dr. Barstow. The last time you played doctor like this, you walked around with a hairline fracture of your leg for a week before you finally gave up the ghost and went to the ER."

"I was a little stubborn about that, and as I recall, the injury marked the end of my basketball career."

She looked at him askance. "Basketball? You haven't played basketball since college. You injured your leg playing tennis."

"Oh, yeah."

She took a few steps closer to straighten the blanket that had slipped off to the side and was now half on the floor. When Annette raised her eyes, she noticed much of his normally rosy complexion had faded, leaving his face the color of a rice cake. She also observed a barely noticeable quivering of his lips.

"How's your headache, any better?" she asked him.

"Not really. I took some aspirin before, but it's not helping too much. At least I finally got rid of those awful hiccups."

"Aspirin? Where did you get aspirin from? We have kids. We don't have any aspirin in this house. Are you sure it wasn't Tylenol?"

"Yeah...I meant Tylenol."

Annette was about to renew her plea that he allow her to take him to the emergency room when she noticed his eyes had suddenly become vacant and his gaze was aimless.

"John?" He didn't respond. "John," she repeated laying her hand on his shoulder and giving him a gentle shake.

All at once, his right arm stiffened and then locked in a fully extended position. A high-pitched wail escaped his lips as his body pushed to the left, and he began wildly shaking and shuddering. Having grown up with a younger brother who suffered from epilepsy, Annette knew a seizure when she saw one.

She reached for his shoulders to prevent him from falling off the lounger. Keeping his head turned sideways to guard against him aspirating his own saliva, she attempted to pull her phone from her pocket. John's torso twisted more violently, forcing her to struggle to keep him upright. A pool of saliva bubbled at the right corner of his mouth, while his entire body was now jerking as if a powerful pulse of electricity was running through him. Checking his breathing again, Annette could see and hear him sucking in sporadic breaths. His lips were mildly blue. She knew trying to communicate with him would be futile.

Finally, she was able to position him in a way that allowed her to yank her phone out of her pocket. In order to make the call, she slowly eased up on her grip, lowered the footrest, and allowed him to roll toward her. She did what she could to support him, but at best, it was a controlled topple. When she again had control of him, she used her sleeve to dab the saliva from under his mouth.

His seizure showed no signs of abating. Managing to turn him on his side, she passed her right arm around his back and shoulder. With her opposite hand she dialed 9-1-1. Frightened down to her fingertips, she managed to maintain her composure long enough to answer the dispatcher's questions. He assured her a rescue unit was on the way, and she could expect the paramedics to arrive in about ten minutes. Instead of staying on the line as the dispatcher requested, Annette tossed the phone on the floor and turned her entire attention toward assisting John. Over the next few minutes, his seizure slowly began to subside. When she heard the doorbell, she ran to the front door and escorted the two paramedics to the patio.

"Does he have a history of seizures?" the first one to reach him asked.

"No, but he's been pretty sick the last few days."

They continued to work while they asked Annette questions. In very short order, the paramedics had prepared John for an urgent transfer. The moment the IV was in, they gave him two antiseizure medications. They snapped the stretcher to its upright position and rechecked his vital signs. With Annette at the side of the stretcher holding John's hand, they hurried out of the house.

Chapter 17

Jack exited the Beltway and followed the signs for arrivals at Washington National Airport. As he pulled up to the curb in front of Terminal Two, he began scanning the area, hoping to spot Madison. To his delight, he saw her at once, wheeling her suitcase past the head of a very long taxi line. He stepped out of his van and waved to her over the top of the hood. She spotted him, returned the wave, and headed his way. After a long hug, he tossed her bag in the back of the van.

Having curved facial features, the neck of a gymnast and being trimly toned, Madison was a stylish, eye-catching woman whose appearance had not caught up to her years. She and Jack had first met at Shand's Hospital at the University of Florida twenty years earlier when she was a junior medical student rotating on neurology and he was the chief resident. Their relationship had been professional and cordial until the end of her rotation. For reasons entirely unrelated to her performance and unbeknownst to Jack, she received a failing grade. It was her erroneous but unshakable belief that Jack was the one directly responsible for the unsatisfactory review.

Despite his insistence to the contrary, she'd clung to her conviction that he'd submarined her. After an Olympian effort to right the ship, Jack eventually accepted he'd never change her mind. At that point, he was convinced she didn't care to be bothered with the truth, and he gave up. Eventually, they went their separate ways, both being pleased by the prospect of never seeing the other again.

Years later, Madison had learned that it was her ex-husband, also a physician, who had used his influence to mastermind the scheme that resulted in her failing review in her neurology rotation. By pure serendipity, Jack and Madison's paths crossed again ten years later when they were both asked to consult on an enigmatic epidemic of cases in Florida affecting pregnant women. It was an uncomfortable situation for them both, but under the circumstances, they agreed to put their rocky past aside and work together civilly to find a cure for gestational neuropathic syndrome.

Owing to the passage of time and changing circumstances, their new relationship was a distinct departure from the first. As the days turned into weeks, it evolved from polite and platonic to something more serious. Madison developed a strong interest in elusive diagnoses, and although she was principally a perinatologist by training, she'd joined Jack as a consultant on several perplexing new cases. Eventually, after being offered a prominent position at Ohio Children's Hospital, she'd left Florida and moved to Columbus.

"How was your flight?" he asked her, as he maneuvered the van across two lanes of slow-moving traffic toward the airport exit.

"A little too bumpy for me."

"And how's Moose?"

"That slobber-puss of a dog that you're attached to at the hip is fine. My cousin moved in and is taking good care of him. She couldn't believe you left Columbus without him. She didn't know how either of you would deal with the separation anxiety," she answered with a chuckle. "I thought Anise was coming with you to pick me up."

He cleared his throat. "There's been an unexpected development that I need to talk to you about."

"Is she okay?"

"Anise is fine. It's Nicole. She was admitted to the hospital today. It looks like she's probably got viral encephalitis."

"I'm so sorry to hear that, Jack. How long has she been sick?"

"About a week."

"Just how serious is it?"

"She had a seizure and was admitted to a critical care area."

"When did you hear about all this?"

"I was on the Penn Turnpike about two hours out of DC when I checked in with Anise and she told me what was going on. Nicole kept insisting she just had a bad flu. I was concerned by Anise's description of her symptoms, but when I got to Washington and saw her, she was a lot sicker than I imagined."

"Anise must be a wreck. She and Nicole have such a close relationship. How's she doing?"

"Not well. She's devastated."

"Did you speak with Nicole's physician?"

"I met with her at the hospital a few hours ago. Her name's Kristin Hartzell. She works for Marsh Technologies, the same company that employs Nicole. As it turns out, Nicole's the second Marsh employee who's been admitted with a working diagnosis of encephalitis in the last twenty-four hours"

"And what's your role going to be in all this?"

"It seems Nicole asked Dr. Hartzell to keep me fully apprised of her condition."

"I'm a little surprised you didn't offer to get involved in a more hands-on way."

"I did my best to keep our conversation professional, and I was particularly careful not to come across as overly pushy."

An intrigued look came over Madison's face. "How do you think Dr. Hartzell interpreted keeping you apprised? Does that mean as a family member, as a physician, or as a neurologist of national prominence who just happens to be an expert in elusive diagnoses?"

"I'm not sure."

"Hypothetically speaking, what's your plan if she asks you to officially consult on the cases?"

"I don't know, nor do I see any reason to get ahead of myself or Dr. Hartzell for that matter."

She leaned over and placed her hand on his shoulder. "Don't get too jumpy, Jack. I'm just teasing you a little. But I think we both know it's not in your DNA to say no to any colleague who asks for help. It's just a matter of time until she finds out who you are—if she hasn't already—and asks you to get involved."

"I'll deal with that if and when it happens."

"It sounds to me like we'll be rescheduling Anise's college tour."

"At least for a few days. I don't see any other option." A constellation of brake lights lit up the road as the traffic suddenly thickened. Jack slowed the van. "Are you hungry?"

"I could eat," she answered.

"Good. I made a reservation at an Italian restaurant in Foggy Bottom."

"Sounds good, but how about making a quick stop at the Lincoln Memorial first?"

Jack shook his head, unsurprised by her request. Since college, Madison had been an avid traveler of the United States. The grandeur of the brilliantly illuminated Lincoln Memorial at night had remained one of her perennial favorites.

"It might not be a bad idea for me to reach out to Anise," Madison suggested. "I think having leukemia gives me a perspective that might help her cope with the current situation. What do you think?"

"I think that's an excellent idea."

Madison leaned forward and lowered the volume of the music. "When the right time presents itself, I'll broach the topic. Anise is a bright kid, mature beyond her years, but she can be more willful and determined than a salmon swimming upstream—a character trait she no doubt inherited from her father."

"Thank you…I think. I'm sure it'll help if you speak with her," he said, deciding not to mention his similar conversation with Anise. It seemed axiomatic to Jack that if Madison reached out to her, the conversation would be a good start as a relationship builder.

Twenty minutes later they arrived at the monument. Jack got

lucky and found a convenient place to park the van. They walked past the reflecting pool and up the first set of granite steps to the monument's plaza and then up the final steps to the central chamber. Approaching the sculpture of Lincoln deep in contemplation, Jack saw the awe in Madison's eyes. He said nothing, allowing her to take in the stateliness and solemnity of her surroundings.

After a few minutes, they moved on to the north and south chambers. When Madison was ready, she gave Jack the word, and they descended the steps, returned to the van, and drove to the restaurant. Their meal was leisurely and deliciously prepared. Jack did his best to unwind from his trying day, but he couldn't find a way to completely dismiss his uneasy feelings regarding the uncertainties of what the future might hold for both Anise and Nicole.

The combination of the late hour and the Barolo wine they'd enjoyed with dinner left Jack and Madison exhausted. They went straight from the restaurant to the Hay-Adams Hotel, checked in, and headed up to their room. A half hour later, they were both asleep.

Chapter 18

Being in a heavy slumber, the sound of his cell phone startled Jack to where he practically toppled out of bed. He directed a flailing hand to the top of the nightstand until his sleep-filled eyes finally helped him grab his phone. He had a pretty good suspicion who was calling and why. It was ten minutes to one.

"Jack, it's Kristin Hartzell. I apologize for the hour, but Nicole's not doing well, and I thought you'd want to know about it sooner rather than later."

"There's no need to apologize. I appreciate you calling. What's going on?"

"She's having more seizures and increasing respiratory distress. We're doing our best to treat both problems, but we've only been partially successful, and I'm afraid we're running out of options. It looks like we're going to have to put her on a ventilator."

"I'll head into the hospital now. Does Anise know what's going on?"

"Not yet. Seeing how fragile she's becoming, I thought it might be better if she heard this latest development from you, especially if we wind up having to intubate Nicole and put her on a ventilator."

"It's probably a better idea if I call Anise from the hospital after I have a clearer idea of how Nicole's doing."

"That makes sense. I'll see you in a little while…and thanks, Jack."

He looked over at Madison who was wide awake and leaning against the upholstered headboard with her eyes locked on him.

"That didn't sound good."

"Nicole's having seizures and may need to be put on a vent," he said, throwing his legs over the side of the bed.

"Do you want me to come with you?"

"No. You've had a hell of a long day. Try and go back to sleep," he suggested, leaning back over and kissing her forehead.

"Okay, but if you need any help with Anise, let me know. I'll go over and get her and bring her to the hospital."

He started toward the bathroom. "Thanks. I may take you up on that." Ten minutes later, he was dressed and heading out of their suite. It took him only ten minutes to drive to the hospital.

With the first step he took off the elevator, Jack spotted Kristin standing outside of the intermediate care unit. She caught sight of him almost at the same moment, gestured to him to join her, and then escorted him into the unit. A small group of nurses and other healthcare providers stood outside of Nicole's room, creating the type of controlled commotion that always seemed to accompany a patient crisis.

"How's she doing? Jack asked.

"A little worse since we spoke."

"Have you made a final decision about putting her on a vent?"

"I'm leaning heavily in that direction, but I'd like to get the opinion of one of our intensive care specialist before committing to it. He's on his way over now."

Just then, a wiry man wearing oversized rumpled blue scrubs and sporting a crop of peach fuzz on his bony chin approached.

"Thanks for coming over," Kristin said to Arch Britton, the assistant director of all the critical care units. "Let me introduce you to Dr. Jack Wyatt."

"It's nice to meet you," he said, stealing a peek through the doorway at Nicole. "Kristin mentioned you're a physician."

"I am."

"What's your specialty?"

Jack was just about to respond when an anxious-appearing young lady wearing an ID that identified her as an internal medicine resident by the name of Cara West appeared in the doorway.

"Excuse me for interrupting, Dr. Britton, but we need you right now."

"I'll speak with you both in a few minutes," Arch told them, as he quickly moved into the room. A parade of nurses and other healthcare providers rushed in behind him.

Chapter 19

"What's going on?" Arch asked Sarah Cone, the nurse anesthetist, as he hurried to the head of Nicole's bed. Sarah had already placed a bag and plastic mask over her nose and mouth. With each squeeze of the bag, she filled Nicole's lungs with one oxygen-rich breath after another.

"It's not good, boss. Her seizures have gotten a lot worse, and she's not moving much air on her own."

"What's her oxygen saturation been?"

"Terrible. I can't get it any higher than ninety, and her carbon dioxide level's climbing. She's worn out." With a shake of her head, she added, "She's done. She's got no reserve left. I think it's show time." Sarah was an instinctive nurse anesthetist who'd been on staff at the Infirmary since the day it opened. Arch had worked with her enough to know she was rarely wrong in her patient assessments.

While he was rapidly acquainting himself with the urgency of Nicole's condition, Jack and Kristin slipped into the room and found places against the far wall.

"Do you have a recent set of blood gases on her?" Arch asked Cara.

She handed him a report she'd just printed. "We drew these about five minutes ago."

He glanced at the results. "When was her last chest x-ray, and what did it show?"

"A couple of hours ago. Poor lung expansion and peripheral consolidation on the left. I reviewed it with the radiologist. I have it up on the laptop if you want to have a look at it."

"I trust you" he said. "And the status of her seizure activity?"

"They've been ongoing and difficult to control."

"So what do you think, Cara?"

"I think she needs to be on a vent, sir."

"I agree. Let's get it done," he ordered. "Are we ready to go?"

"Sarah gave us the vent settings. We're all set."

Arch looked at Sarah. "I assume you have the drugs drawn up."

"Your favorite cocktail—midazolam, etomidate, and succinyl-choline. They're ready to go."

"You double-checked the doses?"

"No," Sarah admitted. "I triple-checked them."

The hint of a grin appeared on his face. "Go ahead and give the midazolam. I'll need a 7- tube."

"Got it right here, boss."

"Bag her a little faster. Let's see if we can get her oxygen satura-tion closer to a hundred percent before we intubate." Thirty seconds passed. "Forget it, I don't like the way her pulse is dropping. Give her the other two drugs. I'm guessing we're about a minute away from a major disaster here." The words were still hanging in the air as Sarah inserted the needles into Nicole's IV port and pushed both meds into her IV line.

"Drugs are in."

As soon as Arch was sure the medications had taken effect, he gently opened Nicole's limp mouth and inserted a laryngoscope. With the help of the special lighted instrument, he swept her tongue to the side—the standard move that gave him a perfect view of her vocal cords, the landmark identifying the entrance to the windpipe.

He held out his right hand. "I'll take the tube." Sarah placed the endotracheal tube in his hand. Gently rotating the tip to the precise position he wanted, he slid it between Nicole's vocal cords and advanced it smoothly down her windpipe. Once it was exactly where he wanted it, Sarah handed him the tubing leading to the ventilator. Arch gently attached it to the end of the tube. Sarah took a few seconds to securely tape it at the corners of Nicole's mouth.

The ventilator began delivering one perfectly timed breath after another. While Sarah was checking the machine's performance, Arch listened to each of Nicole's lungs with the same high-tech stethoscope his parents had given him the day he was accepted to his critical care fellowship.

"Good breath sounds. We're in business," he announced with a measure of relief in his voice. "Her oxygen sat is coming up nicely. Let's get a stat chest x-ray."

"Her blood pressure and pulse are improving, "Cara said.

After Arch checked and rechecked the ventilator settings and assured himself Nicole was stable, he pulled off his latex gloves, tossed them in the trash, and headed for the door.

Just as he was about to step out into the hall, he said, "Let's get things wrapped up in here and get her transferred over to ICU, ASAP. Great job, everybody—thanks."

As he was making his way out of the room, he spotted Kristin and Jack.

"The intubation went fine, but we have no way of knowing how far advanced the encephalitis is, which means we have good reason to still be very worried about her. We'll get her over to the ICU and see how she does. Hopefully, in the next few days we'll be able to identify the precise viral strain that's causing the illness."

"Thanks, Arch. I'll meet you in the ICU in a few minutes. I'm just going to walk Jack out."

He extended his hand to Jack. "It was nice meeting you. I'm familiar with your work. Hopefully, we'll get a chance to talk when the smoke clears a little."

"I'll look forward to it."

Kristin escorted Jack out of the unit and toward the elevator.

"In addition to our own lab, we're sending spinal fluid and blood to a state-of-the-art viral lab the military runs over at Fort Detrick.

For now, there's not much else I can think of to do, other than let's keep our fingers crossed."

"I agree. Please call me if there are any changes."

Consumed by a mixture of exhaustion and despair, Jack rode the elevator down to the lobby with the plan of calling Anise from the van. He wasted no time heading across the lobby toward the exit. He was just about to leave the hospital when his phone rang. He glanced at the caller ID. He assumed Madison was calling, but it was Kristin. His throat squeezed as he prayed she wasn't calling to tell him know that Nicole had taken yet another turn for the worse.

"Are you still here?" she asked him, sounding somewhat on the unglued side.

"I'm in the lobby."

"I'm sorry to do this to you, but I really need to speak with you."

"I'll come right back up. I'll meet you outside of the IMCU."

"I'm already heading for the elevator. We can talk in the lobby."

"I'll be here," he told her, feeling the anxiety of the moment building.

Chapter 20

Two minutes later, Kristin was off the elevator and approaching Jack. Due to the hour, there wasn't much activity in the lobby.

"Nicole's condition is unchanged, but there's a new problem that I just learned about that I'd like to discuss with you."

"Of course."

She gestured to a pair of beige accent chairs a few feet away.

As soon as they were seated, she said, "I just received a call from the emergency room." She paused and massaged her brow. "They're presently evaluating three patients with severe neurologic symptoms. I know the physician on duty. She's pretty sharp. She suspects encephalitis in all three cases. She gave me a brief rundown, and the symptom complex is very similar to Nicole's and the other patient I admitted earlier."

"Do they all work at Marsh's headquarters building."

"I'm afraid so. Obviously, this complicates things," she said, exhaling a short breath. "I guess I should stop stalling. I'm afraid I haven't been totally forthcoming with you regarding what Nicole told me. The minute she shared with me that you were a neurologist at the University Hospital Center in Columbus and the director of the Elusive Diagnosis Center...well, I knew exactly who you were.

You see, Jack, I'm quite aware of your outstanding accomplishments in the diagnosis and treatment of obscure illnesses. I was quite in awe of the role you and Madison Shaw played in curing gestational neuropathic syndrome and leukemic malnutrition."

Jack fiddled with his watch band. "We were fortunate to work with some talented and highly dedicated doctors and nurses on those cases. The outcome was a team accomplishment in every sense of the word."

"Your gift for diagnosis may be the only thing that eclipses your humility. Despite appearances, I don't consider myself an alarmist when it comes to the practice of medicine. I've taken care of my fair share of sick patients. Based on what's going on in the ER, I have to assume we're looking at a worst-case scenario, which includes the possibility we're dealing with an untreatable and fatal illness. Add to that, we have no idea how many more cases may come through our doors," she added with more apprehension creeping into her voice. It wasn't difficult for him to deduce where she was headed with their conversation. "I understand that, because of Anise, Nicole still plays an important role in your personal life…and I realize that complicates things, but I still have to ask you if there's any way you'd consider spending a few days with us to officially consult on these cases?"

Just as he was about to respond, Jack caught sight of Anise and Madison coming through the revolving glass doors. He signaled them with a wave of his hand, and they quickly walked over. Both he and Kristin came to their feet.

"What's going on with Mom? How sick is she?"

"She's holding her own, but she's had a few seizures."

"A few? I don't understand," Anise said, standing there looking devastated. "What does all of this…"

"Please try to stay calm. Mom's perfectly stable right now, but Dr. Hartzell had to put her on a ventilator to help her breathe until her seizures are under control." Placing his hands on her shoulders, he went on, "Give me a sec. I'd like to introduce Madison to Dr. Hartzell so the three of us can discuss Mom's condition. Why don't you head upstairs to the waiting room, and we'll meet you there in a few minutes?"

"Do I have to stay in the waiting room? I'd rather sit with Mom. Maybe she'll know I'm there."

Kristin said, "As soon as I get upstairs, I'll check on her and see if it's a good time for you to visit."

Madison walked over to Anise and gave her a hug. "Your mom's going to get better. If there's anything you need…even if it's just to talk, let me know."

"Thanks, Madison. I may take you up on that. I'm sorry I didn't ask how you're feeling. That wasn't very considerate of me. I'm just so focused on Mom."

"As you should be. It's perfectly understandable."

"Are you doing okay…I mean, the leukemia hasn't…?"

"I saw my hematologist last week. She said everything looks great—no sign of even one leukemia cell."

"That's wonderful news. I'm so happy for you."

"Thanks. Now all we have to do is get your mom healthy again." Madison gave Anise another hug. Seeing how hard she was fighting to hold back a new wave of tears, she left her arm around her waist and walked her to the elevators.

Chapter 21

As soon as Anise was on her way up to the fourth floor and Madison had returned, Jack formally introduced her to Kristin.

"I'm sorry we're meeting under such difficult circumstances," Kristin said.

"Hopefully that won't be the case for long. Jack told me he's very impressed with the care you've been giving Nicole."

"Coming from him, that's quite a compliment."

"How did Anise find out what's going on?" he asked.

"She phoned the hospital to check on Nicole. When the nurse filled her in, she tried calling you but couldn't get through. She phoned me, and I told her you were already at the hospital. That's when she insisted on joining you. I managed to persuade her to wait for me, and we came over together in a cab."

Jack moved his gaze to Kristin. "I've filled Madison in on everything we know to this point about Nicole's condition."

"Have there been any new developments besides her seizures?" Madison asked.

"When you and Anise came in, I was just mentioning to Jack that I'd received a call from the ER. It seems they're presently evaluating three patients with neurologic symptoms quite similar to

Nicole's. The physician I spoke with suspects they have encephalitis. She's already sent off complete sets of blood work and has done a spinal tap on each of them. Obviously, they'll require admission to the hospital and further testing. I'm just on my way now to see them."

"So one case of encephalitis has become five," Madison said.

"I'm afraid so. I've already spoken to our nursing supervisor. Our plan is to keep them all together, so we're in the process of setting up a special pod for them in the intermediate care unit." Kristin steadied herself, swapped a ready look with Jack and continued. "You might as well hear this from me, Madison. I just asked Jack if he'd consider spending a few days with us as a consultant. Naturally, we'd be beyond pleased if you'd agree to take on a similar role and be part of our team as well."

"I'm honored you'd ask me."

"Please give some consideration to my request," she said, checking the time. "I should be getting to the ER, and I'm sure you're both anxious to join Anise. Perhaps we can talk later this morning about my proposal."

"That won't be necessary," Madison was quick to reply. "We'd be pleased to do anything we can to help."

Kristin's face instantly filled with joy. "That's…that's wonderful to hear. I…I don't have the first clue how to begin to thank you both. I'll make the arrangements as soon as I can to have you both designated as visiting faculty with full consulting privileges and access to our electronic medical records system."

"That sounds fine," Madison said, turning to Jack. "Why don't you go and meet up with Anise? Since we'll be getting involved, if it's okay with Kristin, I'd like to go with her to the ER to see the new patients."

"It's more than okay with me. Let me make a quick phone call, and we'll go straight over there," she told Madison as she stepped away.

Madison gave Jack's shirt sleeve a quick tug.

"I hope you're not upset that I didn't take Kristin up on her offer for us to take some time to think things over. Since there's no way you'd turn her down, I assumed it would be a giant waste of time."

"Don't worry about it. You did the right thing. Let's hope we get lucky and one of the cultures grows out a virus we can treat."

"Do you think that's likely?"

"Normally I'd say it's probably fifty-fifty, but I think there's something more than meets the eye about this illness. I've never seen a cluster of encephalitis cases like this unless there was an obvious cause, and most of the time those were traceable to either tick or mosquito bites."

"It's almost Thanksgiving, which puts mosquito season largely behind us."

They spotted Kristin heading back toward them.

"All set?" she asked, unbeknownst to her that one of the three patients she was on her way to see in the ER was John Winkler.

"Ready," Madison answered.

"I'll join Anise and catch up with you two in a little while."

Before he'd reached the elevators, Jack's mind was bouncing from one possibility to another. To his dismay, none of them made much sense. He cautioned himself to stay focused and start unraveling the diagnostic dilemma one layer at a time, beginning with what they knew about the disease. He reminded himself that he'd been to this rodeo before, and the keys were to remain patient, never stop thinking, and look at every clue from all angles.

Part II

Chapter 22

FIRST DAY

By the time Jack and Madison got Anise home and had returned to their hotel, it was four a.m. Just like Nicole, the three encephalitis patients in the ER were healthy individuals a week ago who were now seriously ill with a symptom complex consistent with encephalitis.

It wasn't until noon that they returned to the hospital. By that time, the special unit Kristin had talked about establishing for the Marsh patients was up and running. As soon as they entered the intermediate care unit, they spotted her speaking with a group of nurses at the core desk. They waited until she was finished and then joined her. She was slump-shouldered, and her eyelids drooped from extreme fatigue.

"Good afternoon. Did you get any sleep at all?" Madison asked her.

"I'm afraid not. I feel like an intern again. But I survived it once, so I guess I'll just have to survive it again."

"How's Nicole doing?" he asked.

"Holding her own, but certainly no better. We're having a challenging time managing her seizures and her respiratory failure. I don't know when we'll be able to get her off the vent."

"How are the three patients we admitted through the emergency room?" Madison asked.

"Actually, it turned out to be five. Two more employees came in after you guys left. That makes a total of seven encephalitis patients." She added, "The nurses and staff are already referring to them as the 'Marsh patients.'" She made finger quotes as she spoke.

Madison crossed her fingers and held them up. "Hopefully there won't be any more cases."

"I'm afraid that hope is probably in vain," Kristin said. "In the last hour, I've received two calls from outside emergency rooms to advise me they're transferring a Marsh employee to the Infirmary. Both of the attending physicians I spoke with felt encephalitis was the most likely diagnosis."

"Do these new patients have anything in common?" Jack asked.

"Except that they're all Marsh employees, there's no obvious common link. One of the patients is a C-Suite VIP—Oren Severin. Arch Britton's been here all night, struggling to take care of these folks."

"Once we get a detailed history on each of the patients, we'll have a better shot at figuring out if they have a key element in common," Jack said. "What have their major symptoms been?"

"Similar to Nicole, lethargy, headache, and other neurologic symptoms including seizures. The other thing we're fighting is a deterioration in their ability to breathe." Kristin slipped her hands into the pockets of her lab coat. "Now that you two are official consultants, please tell me where you'd like to start."

"Jack and I were just talking about that on the way over. We both think we should do a thorough chart review to familiarize ourselves with everything we know to this point before we make formal rounds."

"The same idea crossed my mind. I've already made arrangements for you both to have complete access to our electronic medical records system. If you'd like, we can go over to the physician charting area now, and I'll give you an orientation to our system and get you started. When you're done, we can meet up and make rounds. In the meantime, I'll sneak up to my office and start on the dozen or so phone calls I need to make."

"That sounds good," Jack said. "What time would you like to make rounds?"

"How about two? We can meet right here."

"That works."

They were just about to make their way to the physician charting area when a jug-eared man of short stature with a stethoscope popping up out of his sports coat pocket joined them.

"Good morning, Kristin," he said, regarding Jack and Madison through the tops of his eyes.

"Elias, I'm glad we ran into you," she said. "I'd like you to meet Drs. Jack Wyatt and Madison Shaw."

"Dr. Elias Rutledge," he said, offering them each a limp-wristed handshake.

"Elias is our chief of internal medicine, and he also serves as the Infirmary's director of medical affairs. I spoke with him earlier and let him know you both have agreed to consult on the encephalitis cases."

With a receding jaw and a cue ball for a scalp in place of hair, Rutledge never missed the opportunity to move center stage and take charge of any meeting he attended. To his credit, he was a knowledgeable physician who took the practice of medicine seriously, but his pompous manner was known to put off his colleagues more often than not.

"Welcome to our hospital. Obviously, your reputation precedes you," he told them in a voice that had an acerbic lilt to it. He absently tapped the tip of his nose a couple of times. "I hope you'll take this in the right spirit, but it's coals to Newcastle having you two join our team. In fact, I was more than a little surprised to learn that Kristin had extended the invitation. We're not exactly a bunch of rookies practicing medicine in some backwoods hospital. We routinely handle some of the toughest cases in DC with great expertise and that would include encephalitis."

"Your hospital is held in very high regard," Jack said, having no problem responding with a sprinkle of implied sarcasm. "Madison and I are looking forward to investigating these cases in the company of such an esteemed medical staff."

"Actually, I'm astonished these cases have stirred up as much hoopla and excitement as they have. I suspect—"

"Elias, I'm sure Jack and Madison understand—"

"As I was saying," he continued as he cast a disapproving glance Kristin's way. "As physicians, we sometimes tend to overthink illness. In these cases, the cause is clearly viral. We haven't identified the strain yet, but with the expert lab facilities we have at our disposal, I expect we'll have an accurate diagnosis within a few days." He shrugged his shoulders and added, "Once we've identified the offending virus…well, the matter's out of our hands."

"Out of our hands?" Kristin asked.

"Yes, of course. Either the strain is treatable by the antiviral medications we have available to us or it's not." He shifted his attention to Jack. "I was informed that one of the patients is your ex-wife."

"That's correct. Her name's Nicole Wyatt."

"I hope your personal connection won't cloud your professional objectivity or judgment in any way."

"I'm comfortable I'll be able to maintain an acceptable level of objectivity and professionalism." Knowing Madison's propensity to counterattack without much provocation, especially if the individual slinging the arrows was obviously a self-inflated buffoon, Jack placed a calming hand on her forearm before any verbal gunplay broke out.

"I hope so, Dr. Wyatt, but I guess only time will tell," Rutledge said, lifting the chain that led to his gold pocket watch. He flipped open the lid and carried on with his theatrics by sighing and then shaking his head several times. "I'm late for a rather important meeting. I'm sure we'll have other opportunities to talk." Without waiting for a response, he removed his cell phone from his coat pocket, fixed his eyes on the home screen, and strolled away.

"Is there anything I could say in the way of an apology that would excuse Elias's ill-mannered behavior?" Kristin asked.

"I've had some pretty frosty first meetings, but that may be the new grand champion," Madison said.

"I apologize. I wasn't expecting to see Elias. If it had occurred to me that we might run into him, I would've prepared you by letting you know he can be a little brusque at times and rub people the wrong way."

"I have no trouble believing that," Madison said.

"In his defense…and you may find this hard to believe, but once you get past his haughty, smartest-person-in-the-room persona, he's actually a pretty caring doctor."

"You're correct," Madison said with a skeptical sneer. "I do find that hard to believe." Kristin couldn't contain a grin. "Maybe the next time we meet his disposition will be a little sunnier."

"Madison can be a little direct herself," Jack said to Kristin, adding a wink.

"I love her already. C'mon, I'll get you set up on the medical record system."

In Ohio, Jack and Madison tended to move in civil circles. It wasn't often they encountered professionals who were unmannerly all the way to their fingertips. A couple of Jack's strong suits were diplomacy and forbearance, which rendered him skilled in dealing with ticklish situations. But most people who knew him were astute enough not to confuse his courtesy with weakness.

"It's the room right behind the core desk," she told them, just as her phone rang. She reached into the waist pocket of her lab coat and removed her phone. "I'll meet you over there in a couple of minutes," she said as she stepped away to take the call.

"Kristin seems to be a very conscientious physician," Jack said, "but I expect things may get a lot more tense and frustrating before they get better."

"What is it that you're trying to say, Jack?"

"I'm saying we're probably dealing with a disease that will spell trouble for a lot of patients and healthcare providers. I'm not so sure how well Kristin will hold up under the inevitable stress of the situation."

"I'm surprised to hear you say that."

"You obviously disagree."

"Yeah. It's just a first impression, but she strikes me as the kind of woman who has it in her to knock it out of the park whatever the situation is that she faced with."

Chapter 23

Adrift in thoughts unrelated to work, Erik Brickhill walked east on Constitution Avenue until he reached the entrance to the Tidal Basin Loop Trail. It was a sunshiny afternoon with just a few puffy clouds wandering aimlessly across the eastern sky. Erik was a firm believer in using his afternoon off for stress reduction. He enjoyed bouldering, sailplaning, and reading in Woodley Park, but his preferred way of recharging his stress-resilience battery was taking long, brisk walks. He had several routes that he tended to repeat, but oftentimes he just set out and invented his path as he went along.

The historic two-mile Tidal Basin Loop Trail granted access to the monuments memorializing Thomas Jefferson, Martin Luther King Jr., and Franklin Roosevelt. On this particular morning, Erik crossed the Kutz Memorial Bridge and proceeded south, slowing down to appreciate the crabapple trees with their fruit still clinging to their branches and the Jefferson Memorial. As he often did when he reached the FDR Memorial, he stopped for a closer look. He couldn't recall the number of times he'd read Roosevelt's most notable quotes engraved into the granite wall, but it didn't seem to matter, as he always found them inspiring.

"Franklin Delano Roosevelt," came a voice from behind him. It wasn't necessary for him to turn around to put a face to the voice. The distinctive timbre of Regan Cullen's dulcet voice was indelibly fixed in his mind. After a brief but unnatural silence, he did an about-face. She continued, "Obviously, you're an admirer of people who've accomplished great things. FDR was a remarkable leader who believed we define ourselves by our achievements. I couldn't agree more. What about you, Erik. Do you agree?"

Responding to the loaded question, he said, "I guess that depends on the moral and ethical circumstances surrounding those achievements."

"I can't speak for FDR, but I tend to believe great achievements stand on their own. It's a funny thing about moral and ethical imperatives; they're like beauty—they're in the eye of the beholder."

"Without regard for principles and decency, we accomplish nothing," he argued. "But I guess we'll just have to agree to disagree on that one and make it a conversation for another day. Making no effort to hide his annoyance in either voice or manner, Erik added, "I'm off this afternoon. I wasn't aware we had a meeting scheduled."

"Sometimes things come up without warning. I thought it would be better if we discussed the new development at Georgetown Infirmary as soon as possible. I assume your staff has briefed you on your employees who have required admission to the hospital."

"Yes, they have."

"So you're aware that Dr. Hartzell has enlisted the aid of two pretty high-profile consultants."

"If you're referring to Drs. Wyatt and Shaw, I'm aware they'll be joining her team for a short period of time. Is that a problem?"

"To say the least, it certainly came as a surprise to us, yet you seem so blasé about the whole thing."

"It wasn't exactly as if she madly scoured the country searching for help. It's my understanding that, coincidentally, one of the patients is Dr. Wyatt's ex-wife."

"We're aware of that, and perhaps that explains why he and his girlfriend are involved, but it certainly doesn't make us feel any better about the situation."

"I can't imagine why anybody would be frothing at the mouth over Dr. Hartzell's decision, and I won't bother asking why, but it's completely within her authority to assemble whatever medical team she chooses. Her choices regarding patient care decisions don't require board approval."

"I'd hardly refer to Wyatt and Shaw as routine consultants. I'm sure you're aware that they've developed a bit of a rock-star persona in the eyes of the media."

"I think I can save us both a lot of time by simply asking how you'd like me to handle the matter."

"It's not necessary to get so defensive, Erik. I'm only suggesting we exercise a little common sense. As I said, Drs. Wyatt and Shaw know what it's like to be in the national limelight. Simply put, and for reasons that exceed your need to know, that's not the kind of publicity we're looking for."

"Are you suggesting we encourage Dr. Hartzell to thank the doctors and send them on their way?" he asked, letting out a generous breath. "Before you answer that question, let me point out a couple of things. Trying to get rid of them might be a one-way ticket taking you right where you don't want to go with respect to the media. I have no way of knowing how the doctors would react to that, especially since one of the patients is Jack Wyatt's ex. Irrespective of what your particular concerns are, it almost always benefits Marsh Technologies to keep the media at arm's length. At a minimum, getting rid of them for no good reason will raise a lot of the doctors' and nurses' eyebrows. Since neither of us know how much attention these cases might attract in the next several days, showing Drs. Shaw and Wyatt the door could create a firestorm of questions from the media."

"I'm well aware of that—and we're in complete agreement with you. So, for now, we'd simply like you to keep a discreet but careful eye on things and let us know if anything becomes problematic. Seeing as how you're at the top of the organization, you shouldn't have any trouble alerting your staff that you expect to be kept in the loop on things."

"I appreciate your confidence in me," he said with a dose of cynicism. "Was there anything else?"

"As a matter of fact, I do have a question. As you may have surmised, we have no intention of sharing any sensitive information with Dr. Hartzell. But that doesn't mean we're not concerned that, in the course of her medical care of these patients, she could become inquisitive about certain things. My question is, can we count on her to remain a team player?"

"My impression of Dr. Hartzell is that she's an extremely conscientious doctor whose only interest is providing the best possible care to her patients. If you're referring to political issues or something unrelated to her patient care responsibilities, my guess would be she'd have no interest in pursuing anything like that."

"I appreciate your opinion, and I certainly hope you're right. I don't know any of these three physicians personally, but from what I've seen and read, they tend to be inquisitive people, to say the least."

"What's your point?"

"The point is that the finish line may not be in sight just yet, but we're close. Let's both do everything we can to make sure we reach it as planned with no unexpected events."

"I'm sure whatever lengths you've gone to in order to make whatever this problem is go away will be successful."

She grinned. "That had all the sincerity of sending your mortal enemy a Christmas card."

"You could have told me all this on the phone," he informed her with an unsmiling face.

"We're not here to discuss my communication manners. I'm here to educate you. For now, Drs. Shaw and Wyatt are nothing more than a couple of pebbles in our shoe—your main responsibility is keeping it that way," she told him in a flat, calm voice. "You're an enigma wrapped in a mystery, Erik. I just can't seem to figure you out."

"Maybe you should stop trying."

"Maybe I should, but if I were you, I'd get aboard the bus before it runs you over."

"I appreciate the advice, but don't trouble yourself worrying about me."

"I like to worry about things that other people don't care a whit about," she said, turning and taking the first step back in the direction she'd arrived from. "Enjoy the rest of your stroll."

Erik walked over to a water fountain, took a couple of long swallows, and then resumed his walk. He realized he wasn't being nearly effusive enough for Regan Cullen's taste, an attitude that might place him at risk with Marsh's chairman of the board, but for reasons beyond his understanding, he didn't care. It hadn't escaped his attention that he'd decided to do nothing to prevent activity that might be wholly illegal. In spite of the marching orders he'd received, he had to ask himself if he should be proactive in demanding information from Regan.

Having always been comfortable in his own skin, Erik had never turned a blind eye to something he suspected was unholy. He couldn't help but wonder how he'd live with himself if it had been within his power to prevent something catastrophic from happening and he'd knowingly failed to do anything about it.

Chapter 24

As they'd planned, Kristin, Jack, and Madison regrouped in front of the nursing station at two in the afternoon. Looking refreshed, Kristin had traded her wrinkled scrubs for a pressed white coat.

"How did the chart review go?"

"We had a pretty thorough look at all the patients' charts," Jack answered. "As we suspected, their symptoms and diagnostic study results are all pretty similar. What concerns us the most is how rapidly the disease is progressing."

Kristin stated, "To sum up to this point, we've admitted seven Marsh employees who all appear to be suffering from encephalitis, and two more are in the process of being transferred in. They range in age from twenty-two to sixty, and they were all basically in good health before they became ill. One of the women is pregnant, and one gentleman is a well-controlled insulin-dependent diabetic. There's no obvious association that links these individuals together, other than they all work for Marsh. Worth noting is that, in the past couple of months, none of them have traveled to a significant degree, nor have any of them suffered a recurrence of a remote illness that might suggest an autoimmune cause of the encephalitis. To summarize, our working diagnosis is viral encephalitis. Since we're all pretty familiar with the diagnostic workup to this point, I won't review all those results. Is there anything I've omitted or that you'd like to add?"

"What about other cases in the city we might not know about?" Madison asked.

"None that we're aware of. We've made calls to the area hospitals. Apart from the two patients en route to us now, we've received no reports of more cases."

"Jack and I noticed you're ruling out any type of toxic exposure."

"We've either sent or we're in the process of sending blood and urine samples to be tested for toxins known to produce neurologic symptoms. I've gotten back some early results, none of which show any abnormalities. It's not as if they're working in a plant that manufactures pesticides or some other potentially toxic products. Our corporate headquarters is purely an office environment. Over a thousand employees work there. If our problem is some type of harmful exposure, I imagine we'd be seeing a lot more cases." Kristin dug into the top pocket of her lab coat and pulled out a couple of three-by-five cards that she'd been making notes on. After glancing at them briefly, she added, "That's about all I have. Any suggestions about what direction we should take from here?"

Ever the diplomat, Jack spoke up. "I think we need to take a deep breath and think about one thing. All the patients have been ill for about a week. It's not surprising we don't have any meaningful answers yet. There is a mountain of possibilities, but there's only one thing that I'd say is for sure—at the heart of this disease, there's something tying all the patients together. If this illness is as complex as we all suspect it might be, then we should accept the fact that we need more time to put the pieces together."

"That makes sense—any other thoughts?" she asked. Jack and Madison shook their heads. "In that case, how about making some rounds? I think it's about time you met these folks. Let's start with Kenneth Tolliver. He was one of the later admissions from last night. He got to the unit at about four a.m. His blood pressure keeps dropping, and his urine output has been marginal. His cognitive function has deteriorated in just the few hours since his admission. As Madison may remember from last night, his MRI and spinal tap were normal."

They made their way down the central corridor of the IMCU until they arrived at the entrance to the sixteen-bed pod that had been designated for the Marsh patients. Kristin was about to tap the metal plate to open the sliding glass doors when her phone rang.

She answered it, and after listening for a minute, a frustrated look took over her face.

"Of course, Aaron," she said. "I'm with them right now. We can be there in about five minutes, if that works for you." She ended the call and put her cell phone away. "I'm sorry, but we're going to be delayed for a bit. That was Aaron Steele. He's Marsh's chief legal counsel. He's here this morning attending a meeting and heard about you agreeing to help, and now he wants to meet you to thank you in person. He asked me if the three of us were available." With a conciliatory shoulder shrug, Kristin added, "I'm sure I can come up with some lame excuse to turn him down, but that might not be the best political move. I'm sorry to say this, but I don't think we should sidestep the meeting."

"We'd be happy to meet with him," Jack said. "It shouldn't delay us too long." He instantly heard Madison clear her throat. He had a very good hunch what was coming.

"Do you need both of us to go?" she asked Kristin directly.

Her request hardly surprised Jack, being well aware of Madison's dislike for anything political, especially gratuitous meetings, and her interest in starting rounds. Jack smiled inwardly.

"That shouldn't be a problem. I'll tell Aaron you're involved with a patient care matter. I think Jack and I should be able to muddle through this."

Turning to him, Madison asked, "Do you mind if I pass on the meeting?"

"Would it matter if I did?"

She eyed him silently, and he grinned.

"Just kidding. I don't mind," he assured her.

"While Jack and I are meeting with Aaron, you might want to

take a look at Lori Somersby," Kristin suggested. "She was the patient who came in a few hours before Nicole. She's in her first trimester of an uneventful pregnancy. We have a small OB service here at the Infirmary, but we don't generally handle any high-risk obstetric patients. With your background in perinatology, I'd sure like to get your opinion. If you're up for it, I'll arrange to get you a fetal stethoscope and an ultrasound machine."

"I'd be happy to see her."

"Great. She's in 4004. Jack and I should be back here in about half an hour, and hopefully we'll finally be able to get started on rounds. I guess this is the price you pay for being a doctor employed by big business." They shared a chuckle. "If it looks like things are going to drag on any longer than that, I'll give you a call."

"Sounds good," Madison said as she started back to the chart room to have another look at Lori's medical record before going to see her.

Chapter 25

Lori Somersby had accepted a job at Marsh Technologies when she was nearing the completion of her master's degree in electrical engineering. She felt the organization had always treated her fairly, having advanced her up the ranks faster than most of her colleagues. In addition to being innovative and an excellent communicator, her work product was consistently on point.

When Madison finished her chart review, she made her way to Lori's room. As she approached the bedside, she was most struck by Lori's washed-out complexion, lack of facial animation, and the drops of perspiration that speckled her forehead and the bridge of her nose. From a neurologic standpoint she was in a state of pre-coma, spending almost the entire day sleeping and being extremely slow to respond to any form of stimuli. Fortunately, her respiratory status had remained acceptable, precluding the need to place her on a ventilator. As was the case with Nicole, her symptoms and diagnostic studies were compatible with encephalitis.

Madison's eyes scanned each of the digital monitors. Lori's blood pressure and pulse, the oxygen content of her blood, and her respiratory rate were in acceptable ranges, although only just. She wasted no time in beginning her physical examination. As she was carefully palpating Lori's abdomen, a nurses' aide entered the room, rolling a cart carrying a fetal ultrasound machine and a stethoscope.

"Where would you like the cart, Dr. Shaw?"

"If you could please leave it right there on the other side of the bed, that would be great…and thanks."

When Madison completed her examination, she turned on the ultrasound machine and waited for it to boot up. She took her time obtaining all the views and measurements necessary to assure nothing escaped her attention. To her relief, there were no significant abnormalities she could see that would put Lori's unborn baby girl at risk. In addition to the ultrasound, Madison planned on ordering other key tests to complete her fetal evaluation. She was finishing up the ultrasound when she heard the door open. A smartly dressed woman with porcine eyes and tapered fingers entered the room.

"Good morning. My name's Gretchen Chan. I'm Lori's wife. I don't think we've met, although I suspect you must be Dr. Shaw. Lori's nurse mentioned I'd probably find you here."

"It's a pleasure to meet you."

Gretchen parked her rolling computer case against the wall and then walked over to the bedside.

"So tell me, how are mom and baby doing?" Madison could read in her eyes that Gretchen was careworn and doing her best not to become unhinged.

"The baby's feeling the stress of Lori's illness, but I'd say, based on the limited information I have, at least for the moment, she's in no immediate danger. That being said, there are some other tests I'd like to do. I'm sure you understand that, when we're dealing with a fetus, things can change very quickly."

"Even though it comes with some cautions, it's nice to get a piece of good news."

"Do you mind if I ask you a few questions?" Madison inquired.

"Of course not."

"How long have you known Lori?"

"Seven years."

"And how would you characterize her general health?"

"On a scale of one to ten, I'd say she's a solid eleven. In fact, until now, I can't remember a single day that she's ever really been ill." Picking up a brush from the nightstand, Gretchen began to gently brush Lori's long brown hair.

"Has she had any difficulty with the pregnancy?"

"She had some nausea early on that soured her mood and made her a bear to live with, but other than that, I'd say she's done well," she said as she plucked a couple of clumps of loose stands from the brush and tossed them in a wastebasket.

"I've had a thorough look at Lori's chart, and I know you've already spoken to Dr. Hartzell and some of the other consultants in detail, so I won't ask you to go over her entire illness. But if there's there anything else you can remember that was out of the ordinary, even if it doesn't seem important, I'd like to hear about it."

Gretchen took a few moments to ponder the question.

"If you phrase the question like that, there was one thing that I don't think I mentioned to Dr. Hartzell or any of the other physicians. I doubt it's important, but I'm happy to share it with you if you'd like."

"I would."

"It was the second day of her illness. She wasn't feeling great by any stretch of the imagination, but she wanted to go out for a quick lunch. I didn't think it was such a hot idea, but anybody who knows Lori knows she can be more persuasive than a starving life insurance salesman. So I caved in. We were about halfway to the restaurant when I pulled up to a red light. After a few seconds, she asked me why I was still stopped when the light was green. At first, I thought she was kidding, but when she insisted, I dismissed it as due to the headache and mild blurred vision she'd told me about earlier that day. She did the same thing when we were on our way home too. I guess over the next couple of days, when she was becoming more ill, I just kind of forgot about it."

"For genetic reasons, women get the more common forms of color blindness much less frequently than men. Do you know if Lori has ever been diagnosed with a visual color deficiency?"

"She never mentioned it, and she's not one to hold things back or keep secrets. If she knew she had a form of color blindness, she would've told me. I've been driving with her for as long as I've known her, and I've never noticed a problem." She paused for a few moments and then inquired, "I know you can't be completely certain about a lot of things, but can you at least give me some idea of what the next few days may be like for her?"

"I wish I could, but so much depends on us finding the specific cause of the illness. The only way to do that is for us to stay focused on how the patients are responding to our treatment."

"I'm a district court judge, Dr. Shaw. I know how to be blunt. So if you'll allow me to be direct, what are Lori's chances of surviving the illness?"

"If we can find an effective treatment, I'd say her chances are good. If we can't, the possibilities range from complete recovery to partial recuperation with neurologic impairment all the way to losing her."

With her eyes cast downward, she said, "I guess I kind of suspected that's what your answer would be."

"Things could change from hour to hour. We always tell our patients' families to try and be patient, but I'm not sure I can tell you how to accomplish that."

"I'll be okay. To use a trite expression, I'm hoping for the best but preparing for the worst." She glanced over at Lori and said in a voice that trailed off, "Lori's the love of my life, Dr. Shaw, and our baby's something we've been praying about for the last few years."

Madison moved toward the middle of the room to get closer to Gretchen.

"I promise you that I'll do everything in my power to get Lori and the baby through this." Madison was completely sincere in her pledge to Gretchen but well aware that it would probably do little to boost her optimism. "I'll stop back later today. I'd like to introduce you to Dr. Wyatt. He'll be consulting on Lori's case also."

"Thank you, Doctor. I look forward to meeting him."

Madison stepped out into the hall.

She believed she was as practiced as any physician when it came to the near-impossible task of keeping your personal emotions separate from your clinical responsibilities. She understood the time-honored precept that a physician had to be objective to be an effective healer. Based on her own experience both as a doctor and as a patient being treated for leukemia, she was no longer convinced of its dogma. Gretchen was suffering. How could anybody, even someone with an MD after their name, who had a heart in their chest completely sweep their personal emotions aside.

As Madison walked toward the core desk, she spotted Kristin and Jack.

"How was your meeting?"

"Interesting," Jack answered with a cryptic look on his face. Madison took that as her invitation to ask him all about it later.

"Did you get a chance to see Lori?" Kristin asked.

"I just left her room a couple of minutes ago. Unfortunately, I didn't learn much more than I'd already discovered when I reviewed her chart. The baby's holding her own, but I don't know how long that will be the case. Obviously, if Mom continues to decline, especially at the rate she is, fetal distress is inevitable. I met Lori's wife, who's quite bright and seems to have a realistic idea of what they're up against."

Kristin said, "I'm hoping, after we've rounded on all the patients, we'll have a better idea of what's going on. Somehow, we have to figure out the best next step for these folks."

"So which patient would you like to start with?" Madison asked.

"I separated them into three groups based on the severity of their illness. John Winkler clearly falls in the most critically ill group, so I suggest we start with him."

As they started down the hallway, Jack thought about what he'd intentionally left unsaid. He knew the next three days would be critical. It would take time to get the majority of the test results back from the lab. If they were negative, it would mean a less likely chance of being able to successfully treat the disease. By three days from now, Nicole and the other patients could deteriorate to a point where they'd be basically untreatable. Well aware that such an occurrence would seal their fates, Jack shuddered at the thought.

Chapter 26

SECOND DAY

As he did every morning, Ed Terry threw back his down comforter at precisely five a.m. After wolfing down a larger breakfast than most people would eat, he took his standard poodle, Fifi, for her daily one-hour jaunt along Cardinal Forest Park's extensive network of walking trails. It was the beginning of a breezy day, with the first light of dawn filtering through the dense branches of a large stand of ash trees. As she usually did, Fifi stopped every twenty feet or so to do an olfactory exploration of the underbrush that lined many sections of the trail. Owing to the expansive extent of the paths and his preferred early hour, it was uncommon for him to encounter other walkers or joggers.

Ed was a widower with no children who enjoyed his job at the Defense Contract Management Agency. He realized most people would have found the position somewhere between uninteresting and downright boring, but he found it a challenge. Never allowing himself to be lulled into complacency, he enjoyed diving into the details of his projects, scrutinizing and double-checking every line of the many progress reports and contracts he reviewed.

Ever since Oren Severin had shared John Winkler's report with him, he'd devoted a significant amount of time to conducting his own internal investigation. As he'd told Oren, he wasn't going to kick the report upstairs unless he felt it warranted it. The easiest thing he could have done was label it an absurd product of some inventive employee's overactive imagination and drop it in the trash. But Ed was a naturally cautious man, and it was rare for him to dismiss anything out of hand without an overwhelming reason to do so. If there was any chance Winkler had stumbled onto something, and Ed either ignored or missed it, it could turn out to be a blunder of astronomical proportions.

He was about halfway into his walk when he saw a trim woman wearing white athletic gear swinging her arms freely as she race-walked toward him. When she was about ten feet away, she stopped and began to run in place. A moment later she looked up and smiled at him. He returned the greeting with a smile of his own and moved to the left to pass her.

"Good morning, Mr. Terry." she said as he was going past her.

He stopped and did his best in the limited light to study her face. Unable to recognize her, he instantly found himself at a loss for words.

"Good morning," he said, still struggling to figure out if and when he'd ever met her.

"Enjoying your walk?"

"I am, but I must apologize for not remembering your name. I have a pretty good memory, and generally I don't have too much trouble putting a name to a face. Have we worked together?"

"Not formally. My name's Regan, and I thought you'd be here," she said as she dropped her left hand into her fanny pack. "But I'll tell you something, Ed, in my line of work, you can never be sure of the information you're given, so it's always best to trust but verify." Her hand emerged with a Glock 26 equipped with a magazine extender and a silencer.

"I...I don't have much money," he said with a gasp, feeling his breath catch and his pulse quicken.

"I don't need your money, but I'll take it anyway."

He quickly pulled his brown billfold from his pocket and held it up.

"Please don't hurt me," he said as he tossed it at her feet. Having been raised in Chicago and then going off to college and graduate school in Philadelphia, he was familiar with the best way of saving your life if you became the victim of a mugging. "I'll just go on my way. I'll never report this or tell a soul about you."

"I believe you," Regan said, as she raised the Glock level with his heart and discharged two rounds into his left chest. Both penetrated the main chambers of his heart.

His legs instantly folded under him. From the incline of the trail, he toppled forward, landing a couple of feet from her with his arms raised above his head. Having not a scintilla of doubt that he was dead, she eased forward and kneeled down beside him in a baseball catcher crouch. Within a few seconds, a frothy mixture of air and blood bubbled between a pair of shattered ribs, staining his yellow sweatshirt. She gazed at the mark for a few moments before tilting her head to the side. She was struck by how much the stain reminded her of a silhouette of a line of skyscrapers.

Fifi frantically ran back and forth across Ed's lifeless body, stopping to sniff and bark with each pass she made. Regan reached down, scooped up the wallet, and slipped it into her fanny pack. Glancing at him a final time, a random expression occupied her face. Taking a generous breath of the morning's cool, soothing air, she reached down and picked up the handle of the dog's leash. Taking a final look around, she confirmed there was nobody in sight.

"Don't be sad, girl," she said gently stroking the top of Fifi's head. "There's nothing to worry about. I've already got a nice new family picked out for you." She took a moment to move the Niagara Falls cap she was wearing a half-turn so the visor was pointing backward, and with her new friend in tow, she started back to the park's entrance.

Chapter 27

It was a few minutes past two in the afternoon when Kristin stepped off the elevator on the second floor of Marsh's Technologies' four-hundred-thirty-thousand-square-foot corporate headquarters. The second floor was the centerpiece of the magnificent structure and contained the executive conference room and the C-suite's swanky offices.

Still a little uncertain as to why she'd been summoned to another meeting with Aaron Steele, she made her way down the broad corridor with its walls adorned with plaques, awards, and framed certificates recognizing Marsh for its continued excellence in the defense contract industry. Kristin had worked with Steele on several projects since being hired at Marsh and was well acquainted with his leadership style. Her opinion of him was mixed, finding him to be a grandstander of sorts who oftentimes lacked sincerity but believed he had the insight and eloquence to charm the birds out of the trees. At times, Kristin found him to be more transparent than a mountain lake. Fiercely loyal to the corporation, Steele often resorted to arm-twisting with total impunity, when a more skilled leader would have chosen gentle persuasion.

She entered Steele's outer office and was greeted by a serious-appearing young man. His eyes met Kristin's as he came out from behind his desk.

"Good day, Dr. Hartzell. He's expecting you," he said, escorting her across the room. He stopped in front of the door, knocked once, and opened it.

"Thank you," she told him as she stepped inside.

The expansive office with its glass window wall provided a stirring view of the Pentagon. The grandeur of the room included a walnut conference table with a beveled glass top, plush Saxony carpeting, and handcrafted wall units.

Steele came forward to meet her in the middle of the office.

"Thanks for taking the time to speak with me. Can I offer you something to drink?"

"No, thanks, I'm fine."

He gestured to the conference table on the far side of his office. Once Kristin was seated, he took the high back chair directly across from her.

"How are our patients doing?"

"I wish I could say they were doing better. The infection seems to be intensifying, which is obviously taking an extreme toll on them."

"I'm so sorry to hear that. The reports we've been receiving haven't been very encouraging. Is there a reasonable chance they'll pull through?"

"We certainly hope so. We'll just have to wait and see."

With clasped hands and a measured sigh, he said, "I'm sure I don't have to tell you that this…this tragic situation has hit us all like a runaway freight train. We consider all our employees to be like family, and I promise you that you'll be provided with every resource you need to help them get through this. That promise comes directly from the top…and I don't mean Erik Brickhill, I mean the chairman of the board."

"I never doubted for a moment we'd have the full support of the executive team. I'm very aware of their commitment to the health-care needs of our employees."

"That's certainly gratifying to hear, Kristin. I'm sure you know just how much we value you as an integral part of the team."

"I appreciate those kind words."

A solemn look emerged on his face, prompting Kristin to suspect the effusive opening to their meeting was about to end and that he was ready to broach the reason he'd summoned her to his throne room.

"I thought it was about time you and I had a little chat in private. I know it's probably not necessary, but during these tense and difficult times…well, I just want to make sure we touch every base and that we're singing from the same hymn book."

"Of course, Aaron."

"From what I understand…and please correct me if I'm wrong, at the present time, there's no reason to suspect Marsh was negligent or responsible in any way for how these folks contracting this terrible disease." He paused, picked up his fountain pen, and slid a white legal pad closer to him. "Would you agree with that?"

"Since we don't know the specific cause of the encephalitis yet, the most I can say is that there's no evidence at this time to suggest we did something negligent to cause the illness. The other thing worth mentioning is that, while viral encephalitis is our working diagnosis, we could be completely wrong. That's why we can't and haven't closed the door on other possible diagnoses."

"I wasn't aware of that. I assumed your team was convinced they had the correct diagnosis, and you were focusing on finding out which virus was the culprit so you could treat it."

"That's not exactly the case."

He forced an uneasy smile to his face and then averted his eyes momentarily. Kristin was surprised he'd done such a poor job of disguising his displeasure.

"Of course, I'll leave the medical matters to you, but please assure me that the doctors at the Infirmary are doing everything in their power to help these employees."

"You have my word," she told him again, wondering when the fluff would end and he'd get to what was really on his mind.

"Please understand, I'm not trying to cloud or interfere with the medical answers your team is so diligently pursuing, but none of us operate in a silo, and we can't lose sight of the fact that we have the company's good name and future to consider."

"I'm focused on my patients, Aaron. I assure you, none of our professional activities impact the company's good name," she said with a purposeful tilt of her head.

"Your refreshing idealism may be a little naïve. And while it's commendable, it may not reflect the reality of being a multi-billion-dollar defense contractor."

"Why don't you educate me?"

"While we'll remain optimistic that these folks will pull through, we must consider how we'll handle things if the situation doesn't turn out that way. It doesn't take a PhD in public relations to see that it's quite possible that we're going to be facing some very tough questions from the media."

"That would seem only natural, but if we answer them honestly, I don't see why there'd be a problem. Right now, our working diagnosis is encephalitis. It's our job to treat it. No doctor or hospital in the world can claim they cure every illness."

"There've already been a few stories in the papers and on one on TV. With the number of affected employees increasing, we have to assume media interest will increase as well. We're comfortable the information didn't come from Marsh or the Infirmary, but with so many family members involved…well it's not surprising that somebody spoke with the media."

"I agree; that eventuality seems inevitable."

"Which brings me to a very important point. Because of the nature of the illness, we feel new medical information is going to become available…maybe even on a daily basis." He stood up, walked around to the other side of the conference table, and sat down in the chair next to hers. He crossed his legs at the ankles. "We feel the best way to approach the media is not to release any medical information unless it's been screened first by our media consultants."

"As a physician, I don't discuss the details of my patients' conditions with the media. It's part of an oath I took at my med school graduation," she added with a cutting tone to her voice. "I'm happy to leave dealing with the media to you and your team."

"I'm aware of your Hippocratic oath, Kristin, and I'm not trying to offend you, but we have every reason to be concerned. This company's reputation could be unjustifiably and unfairly tarnished. Or worse."

"At the risk of repeating myself, as long as we're honest and open, we shouldn't have anything to worry about. And, just to put you at ease, if there is an information leak or indiscreet public comment, it won't come from me."

"I'm not suggesting you or any other doctor or nurse would intentionally say something embarrassing or harmful. But don't believe for a moment that an innocuous comment can't be manipulated by the media and misconstrued by the public. Sometimes the mere appearance of impropriety can cause untold problems for an organization."

Kristin failed to see how she could make herself any clearer and was fast running out of patience. She'd heard enough of his diatribe, and since their conversation was going nowhere, she was more than ready to put an end to it.

"I fully understand what you're saying, Aaron, but I can't be a party to any intentional concealment of the facts or alternative versions of the truth. For me, that would cross a red line."

"Nor would we ask you to. I assure you, this company's reputation has been built on a solid bedrock of transparency, integrity, and accountability. We would never violate any of those core principals, nor would we expect any of our team members to. That's all I'm trying to tell you," he added before falling silent.

A few moments passed and Kristin stood up. Aaron waited a few seconds before coming to his feet. She got the feeling he wasn't used to people getting up from their chairs before he did.

"Thanks for spending these few minutes with me," he told her in a cultured voice. He escorted through his outer office and down the hall to the elevators. "I'll let the appropriate folks know we chatted and that we're on the same page regarding how to handle these delicate matters." The annoying grin on his face seemed to be glued in place. "If there's anything more you'd like to discuss, please feel free to stop by. You know my policy." Kristin had no idea what he was referring to but nodded her head as if she did. "My door's always open."

On her way down to the lobby, her mind stayed focused on their conversation. Perhaps she could be counted among Marsh's more naïve employees, but she'd have to be downright gullible to think that Aaron's sole purpose for inviting her to his office for a chat was purely a formality to remind her of the importance of the company's image. Her inner voice was telling her she'd just been put on notice as to how the C-suite expected her to conduct herself.

At the same time Kristin was reaching the lobby, Aaron was removing his cell phone from the inside pocket of his double-breasted blue blazer.

"She just left."

"And?" the man asked.

"I'm unconvinced she understands the sensitivity of the situation or the need for complete discretion."

"But can she be trusted not to take matters to the next level?"

"Her loyalty is clearly to her patients and her profession. I don't think she's interested in painting outside of those lines."

"Concern has been raised that things will be made considerably more difficult now that Drs. Wyatt and Shaw are part of the physician team."

"I think that remains to be seen. They're here to help with the medical issues. If they stay in that silo, it's quite possible they could unwittingly assist us."

"I assume you were careful not to raise any suspicions with Dr. Hartzell."

"I doubt she has the insight to suspect that our little chat was anything more than a polite, professional briefing."

"Perhaps you underestimate her."

"I don't think so, but rest assured that I'll be monitoring things very closely in the days to come. If I've taken her too lightly, I'll find out about it soon enough."

"I'm concerned that these physicians are in a position to disrupt our plans. Keep me advised. We may have to arrange for a...a reminder of sorts to make sure we keep control of things."

"I understand."

AARON DIDN'T HAVE the stomach for extreme measures. The man's inference made him cringe. Detached from the moment, he reached for the Rubik's Cube he always kept on his desk. His proficiency at solving it had reached a level that he could practically do it mindlessly. As he worked his way to the final step, he found himself pondering whether Dr. Kristin Hartzell was destined to become the proverbial burr under his saddle.

Chapter 28

THIRD DAY

Madison and Jack were up with the sun, had completed a fast-paced jog around the mall, and were just finishing a light breakfast in their hotel's restaurant.

"Did you call Anise yet?" she asked him.

"I did."

"And?"

"I'd say she's about the same as last night at dinner. We're planning on meeting for lunch and then going to visit Nicole together."

"Did you say anything about her seeing a therapist?"

"A couple of times, but she's dead set against it. For now, I don't feel I should press the point any further."

Jack signed the check and they headed toward the exit.

"Are you feeling the same way I am about rounds yesterday?" Madison asked.

"What do you mean?"

"I'm not sure we learned anything that got us any closer to figuring this illness out. I assume you're still subscribing to your first rule of making a complex diagnosis."

"I've never numbered them. What are you referring to?"

"That nothing really happens until the first decent clue's uncovered."

"That's been my experience as to how it works almost all the time." He pushed back his chair and came to his feet. "C'mon, let's get over to the hospital. I'd like to see Nicole before we meet up with Kristin."

"Sounds good."

It was quarter past seven when Jack and Madison entered the intermediate care unit. The area was waking up, and the bustle of the new shift of nurses, doctors, and other ancillary healthcare providers filled the halls. They hadn't been there more than a minute or so when Nan Case, the nurse who'd been assigned to be the nurse manager of the Marsh patients' pod, approached. Jack and Madison had spoken to her on a couple of occasions and were impressed with her level of skill.

"We admitted two more patients with encephalitis overnight," she told them in just above a whisper. "That brings the total to eleven."

"Marsh employees?" Madison asked. Nan nodded. "How sick are they?"

"I'd say pretty similar to the other patients when they were first admitted."

"And their symptoms?" Jack inquired.

"Also pretty similar to the others," she answered, casting a watchful eye down the hall before going on. "If my nurses weren't already nervous enough, their anxiety levels are really skyrocketing now. All they talk about is how many more encephalitis patients are going to be admitted before all this resolves itself...one way or another."

"Thanks for letting us know," Jack said. "We'll add the new admissions to our patient list. I assume Dr. Hartzell knows."

"I called her at the crack of dawn and let her know." A wary expression appeared on her face. "By the way, Dr. Rutledge also knows. You'll have to excuse me. I have a few meds to give."

"Kristin won't be here until about eight. Why don't you go see

Nicole," Madison suggested. "It's Tuesday morning, and I almost forgot that I'm supposed to check in with my hematologist. I always call her when she's on her way to the hospital. She'll be waiting for my call."

"So this is a routine call?"

"Completely routine but it might take a while, and before you start asking me a million questions, I'm feeling fine."

"How long do you think you'll be?"

"After my virtual appointment, I'd like to make a few calls. Why don't you give me about forty-five minutes?"

"Sounds good, I have some work to catch up on myself. I'll go see Nicole and then probably head downstairs to the medical library," he said, before adding cautiously, "You'd tell me if…if something new was going on…right?"

"I've already promised you that if anything changes with my health, I'll let you know immediately."

"I know, but we could all use a reminder from time to time."

"I think you've used that clever, leadership seminar response in the past."

Madison left the physician charting area and went to the lounge to make her call. Jack took a few minutes to review Nicole's chart before heading to her room. There was no mistaking it—her condition had worsened since yesterday.

The moment he set foot in the room he saw Arch Britton at the bedside examining Nicole. Arch had remained heavily involved in her care from the moment he'd put her on the ventilator and had her transferred to the ICU. Once the special Marsh patient unit had been created, he was comfortable moving her back to her original room. In a short period of time, Jack had gotten to know him fairly well. He was knowledgeable, a skilled practitioner, and exactly the type of physician Jack loved working with on a tough case.

"How's our patient doing?" Jack asked.

"Not very well, I'm afraid. I wish I could say I'm seeing any clinical signs of improvement, but all the evidence is to the contrary. If she hasn't already entered a full-blown tailspin, she's damn close. We're getting close to maxing out on her ventilator settings, and every time we think we've got her seizures under control, she breaks through with a new round. Her lab work's okay, but, unfortunately, every culture and PCR sample we've sent is still negative." He paused and fiddled with his stethoscope, sliding it slowly back and forth across the base of his neck. "It's pretty obvious the antiviral therapy isn't working. Do you or Madison have any revelations to share?"

"I wish we did, but I'm afraid our opinion's not much different than yours. We discussed asking the neurosurgeons to do a brain biopsy to help us make a diagnosis. It's invasive, but it may be the last card we have to play to figure out what's causing the infection."

"You must be reading my diary," Arch said. "When do you think would be the right time to schedule it?"

"It would be a major step with no guarantee it would help. I'm not sure we're quite there yet."

"By the way, how's your daughter doing?"

"Not great. I'm spending as much time with her as I can but nothing I say seems to be making her feel any better."

"Don't give up—we'll eventually get a handle on this thing." He gave Jack a pat on his shoulder and headed toward the door. "I gotta catch up with the residents on teaching rounds. Let's touch base again this afternoon. If there's anything I can do to help...well, you don't have to ask twice."

"Thanks, Arch."

As soon as Arch left the room, Jack sat down and settled his gaze on Nicole. She was heavily sedated, and be it by word or touch, Jack didn't expect her to respond to any stimuli. His mind filled with memories of the years they'd spent together. Divorce had never been the way he wanted to solve the problems between them, but Nicole saw things differently, choosing a legal solution.

Jack suddenly realized he was doing exactly what he'd warned himself not to. His mind flipped back into doctor mode, and he spent the next twenty minutes doing a thorough physical examination. When he was finished, he stepped back and faced the harsh reality that Nicole was showing no evidence she was even in the early phases of recovery. His frustration mounted as he realized he was doing little more than spinning his wheels and that his mind was nothing more than a blank canvas.

It wasn't his ego talking, but he rarely found himself faced with a diagnostic dilemma that he didn't have the first clue as to which way to turn.

Chapter 29

FOURTH DAY

As she did every morning at eight a.m., Kristin turned into the Infirmary's doctors' parking lot and took the first end space she could find. It was a quirky habit she'd acquired when she was training to get her driver's license. She wasn't particularly superstitious, although she'd be the first to admit her minor eccentricities did affect the way she managed many things in both her personal and professional lives.

She was crossing the lobby when she heard a familiar voice calling her name.

"Good morning," Elias said as he caught up to her.

"Good morning."

"I see you're just getting here. I've already been up to the unit, and I'm sorry to report that all eleven patients have deteriorated."

Without slowing her pace, she steadied herself, groaned inwardly, and responded, "We're dealing with severe encephalitis with an unknown cause. I think we both know those are the cases that unfortunately can have a fatal outcome."

"Something I believe I told you from the outset." He halted

briefly before adding, "One thing's for certain, it doesn't appear that the two out-of-town superstars you invited to join our team are saving the day." Kristin would be the first to admit she was not a morning person, which made his signature nasty comments even more annoying than usual. The vision of her father instructing her to always count backward from ten before responding when she felt her anger welling up filled her mind.

"Madison and Jack are excellent physicians with a lot of experience sorting out difficult cases...maybe more than anybody in the country."

"I doubt that's the case, but what's your point?"

"Now's not the time to allow our egos to interfere with our responsibility to our patients."

"Pretty words and nobly stated, but who are we, a bunch of first-year med students?"

As had happened to her on previous occasions, Kristin was quickly becoming convinced that her chances of having a constructive and civil conversation with Elias were about the same as sneaking the dawn past a rooster.

Fighting off the urge to grit her teeth, she said, "Elias, I'm a little pressed for time, so unless you have something of a clinical nature you'd like to discuss about the encephalitis patients, I really should head upstairs and get started on rounds."

With a sweeping gesture of his arm and a major scowl occupying his face, he stormed off in the opposite direction. With a bolt of exasperation coming to rest in her gut, Kristin exhaled a maddened breath and continued across the lobby.

She was just stepping off the elevator when Jack and Madison appeared.

"Good morning," he said.

"Good morning. "How's Anise doing?"

"She seems about the same."

"Hopefully, she just needs a little more time," Kristin said.

They headed down the hall and into the unit. The moment they came through the sliding glass doors, they spotted a commotion outside of Anne Mayor's room. Anne had been one of the patients admitted the day after Nicole. Two years earlier, she had left the academic life at Rensselaer Polytechnic Institute to work for Marsh as a naval architect. Neither employer nor employee ever regretted their mutual decisions.

Jack caught sight of Dr. Ben Thurber, one of the junior attendings, coming toward them. The look on his face spoke volumes.

"Ms. Mayor coded about twenty-five minutes ago. Arch Britton was in the unit when it happened and responded immediately. He's been in there the whole time running the Code Blue."

"How's she doing?" Kristin asked.

"I think they got some response after the first round of drugs. Arch did a pericardiocentesis and drained about fifty milliliters of bloody fluid from around her heart. She improved initially but a few minutes later had another full-blown arrest." Shaking his head slowly, he added, "From what I've heard, she's had no real cardiac function since then. She's only thirty-three and has two kids, so she's getting the full-court press, but I can't imagine they'll persist for much longer."

"Thanks, Ben," Kristin said as they started toward Anne's room to see if they could get a more detailed update on her condition. They were a few steps away when Arch stepped out into the hall. His scrub top was sweat-stained, and his eyes were cast down. The beaten look on his face said it all. When he caught sight of them, he shook his head sluggishly once in each direction and made his way over to join them.

"I'm sorry, guys. I don't think there was any more we could have done. I'm on my way to speak with Anne's husband. I'll give you a call later to go over the details of the code." After an audible sigh from the bottommost part of his lungs, he added, "How am I going to explain to her husband that, for reasons beyond our understanding, his wife and the mother of his children died, and some of the brightest doctors in DC couldn't do a damn thing to prevent it?"

"Do you mind if I go with you?" Kristin asked.

"I don't mind a bit. I'll take all the help I can get."

Kristin shifted her attention to Jack and Madison. "Why don't you guys start making rounds without me? I'll give you a call when we're done speaking with Anne's husband and catch up with you."

"That's fine," Madison assured her.

Kristin was certain the other family members had already learned the first Marsh patient had died. The likelihood that the dynamic between the physicians and the families was about to change dramatically was clear. What she feared most was her suspicion that she was just about to have the first of similar conversations to come with a Marsh patient's family member crushed by the death of their loved one.

Chapter 30

After her disheartening conversation with Anne's husband, Kristin needed a little alone time. She returned to her office to grab a cup of coffee and take a few minutes to compose herself before joining Jack and Madison on rounds. She had just tossed the Styrofoam cup in the trash and was heading out of her office when her hospital phone rang.

"This is Dr. Hartzell. How may I help you?"

"Dr. Hartzell. This is Dr. Alen Benedict calling. I'm the manager of the Special Pathology Laboratory at the United States Army Medical Research Institute of Infectious Diseases at Fort Detrick. How are you this morning?"

"I'm fine," she answered, stopping to take a seat on the corner of her desk. "We've been expecting your call. Thank you so much for getting back to us."

"We were briefed on the urgency of the situation. Marsh Technologies is an important member of our national defense team, and we're pleased to help in any way we can."

"I hope you're calling to tell me you've found something, because we're still scratching our collective heads around here trying to come up with the cause of this terrible illness."

"The best way to put it is that I have both good news and bad news for you." Kristin felt her pulse rate jump. "We've thoroughly evaluated the specimens you sent us from patients Wyatt and Somersby. We used various culture techniques and immunologic studies, and we think we've isolated your pathogen." A sudden surge of relief penetrated to Kristin's marrow, prompting her to subconsciously tighten her grip on her phone. "What you've got is a very unusual strain of adenovirus. We think it's similar in its structure to serotypes 3 and 7. The first time we saw this virus was about six months ago. We've seen a couple more cases since then, but despite our best efforts, we haven't learned too much about it, other than that it can cause significant infections, including encephalitis. We're in the process of setting up a series of studies now, but I'm sorry to tell you it'll be many months before we have any meaningful data on this strain. I wish we could help you more."

"Obviously, that's not what we were hoping for, but it certainly puts us a lot farther down the road than we were before you called. Do you know if any other laboratories have identified the same strain?"

"One in Boston that I know of, and a few others across the country, but I'd say they're no better informed about this new strain than we are."

"Does anybody have a suggestion regarding an effective treatment?"

"I can only tell you what I've heard anecdotally. One physician I spoke with felt cidofovir was the most promising antiviral drug, but his conclusion was based on treating only a couple of patients."

"Were they encephalitis patients?" she asked.

"I don't know the answer to that, but he did tell me the virus was a bad actor."

"I was afraid you'd say that, but at least now we know what we're up against."

"As I said, Dr. Hartzell, I wish we had better news for you. Is there anything else I can do for you?"

"No, not at this time, but I thank you again for getting back to us."

"I'll be sending a written report to you in the next few days. And Dr. Hartzell, good luck. As I said, we're all aware of what's going on at Georgetown Infirmary and hope you can figure out some way to treat the infection. If I come across any new information about the virus, I'll get in touch with you immediately."

Deep in thought, Kristin returned to her desk and sat down. She wanted to think things through for a few minutes before deciding what her next step should be. She understood that Fort Detrick's viral laboratory was a highly sophisticated and state-of-the-art facility, but she was still a little intrigued as to why two other first-rate viral laboratories had analyzed the same patients' specimens and hadn't come up with a thing. A few more minutes passed, and she reached for her phone to call her assistant, Polly.

"Hey. I need you to do something for me."

"Sure. Name it."

"Please email all the members of the physician task group and let them know there will be an emergency meeting this afternoon at five in the fifth-floor conference room."

"What should I put down as the reason?"

"Don't put anything. Also, I'm going to call you back in a little while with the names of a few of the hospital administrators and Marsh execs I'd like you to add to the email list. Oh…and if anybody calls asking what's going on, you don't know anything."

"That's easy. I never do. I'll start the email right now, Dr. Hartzell."

"Better make it an RSVP. If you haven't heard from somebody by three, call them to confirm."

"Will do."

"I know you're the world's most efficient person, but if you have any concern for both of our futures, please don't forget to include Dr. Rutledge."

She giggled. "Not a chance. As my mother used to say, I know my customers."

"I'll get back to you within the hour with the other names."

Kristin's mind filled with troubling questions about the adenovirus. The only encouraging thing she'd gleaned from her conversation with Dr. Benedict was that he didn't know if the new adenovirus strain was uniformly fatal. The question that plagued her the most was now that they knew what was causing the disease, was there any realistic hope of helping the Marsh patients?

Chapter 31

Jack was standing in front of the core desk waiting for Madison when Marietta Chambers, one of the newer nurses to the Infirmary's critical care areas, walked up. Two years out of nursing school, she was confident, reliable, and still eager to learn.

"Excuse me, Dr. Wyatt, but I wonder if you have a minute to have a look at John Winkler." He checked his watch to make sure he still had a little time before Kristin's meeting was scheduled to begin.

"Sure. What's the problem?"

"I took care of him yesterday, and his abdomen was nice and soft. Today it seems like it's swollen and bit tender to palpation."

"Have you noticed anything else?"

"No, just that."

"Okay, let's go take a look."

As they started down the hall, she said, "I know you keep hearing the same thing from most of the nurses…but we're all very concerned that none of the patients seem to be improving. I left the hospital yesterday after spending twelve hours taking care of John. I got back this morning, and he looks worse to me just in that short period of time."

"We changed the antiviral medication he's on last night, and we're hoping that will make a difference. But as you know, it may not be effective. We have no way of knowing yet."

"The word among the nurses is that we're running out of options."

"The plan is to keep pivoting until we find a combination of drugs or other forms of therapy that works." Jack could see in her eyes that she knew his response was vague and generic at best. Jack knew there were few things more important in the care of hospitalized patients than staff morale. The nurses were the primary caregivers and the first line of defense. Keeping them engaged and heartened, while at the same time being forthright with them, was essential.

Jack followed Marietta into the room and went directly to the bedside. John was one of only three Marsh patients who were still breathing on their own. His mental deterioration had been significant, leaving him barely able to respond to questions.

"It's Dr. Wyatt, John. I'm just going to take a minute and check your abdomen."

John's mouth was agape. His eyes were vacant and cavernous. The skin beneath them was paper thin and blood-tinged, as if it was about to peel away on its own.

Jack took some time examining John's belly. It was a little distended but soft and without any palpable masses or suggestion of a large accumulation of fluid. It was clear he didn't have peritonitis.

"I don't think anything serious is going on," he told Marietta. "It's likely his intestines have swelled a little and have stopped contracting. We see it in many disorders, especially in critically ill patients with overwhelming infections. It's the swelling that makes the abdomen look distended. For now, I wouldn't recommend anything except keeping an eye on it."

"Thanks, Dr. Wyatt."

Jack started to pull the blanket up when his eye was caught by the appearance of John's tongue. It was abnormally large, had an odd shine to it, and had lost its normal texture. It was a finding he hadn't noted in any of the other Marsh patients. Intrigued, he took a step closer, his mind flipping into its connect-the-dots mode.

"He's developed glossitis," he said. When an intrigued look landed on her face, he explained, "See how the tongue is inflamed? It can either be an isolated finding or be present as one symptom of a complex illness."

"Do you think it might be important?"

"The problem with a case like this it that a lot of times it's hard to tell at first glance which clinical finding is going to be a key piece of information and which ones aren't."

With an optimistic smile, she held up her crossed fingers. "Let's hope this one is. Thanks for checking his abdomen, Dr. Wyatt."

"Of course. Thanks for bringing it to my attention. Never feel shy about sharing anything that concerns you."

Jack started toward the automatic sliding door. He was just about to exit the room when he stopped, turned around, and set his eyes on John again. He had a sudden feeling that a few of the dots may be lining up. He was more than a little annoyed at himself for missing it. His intrigue mounted like a rogue squall as he made his way back to the bedside.

Easing John's right hand out from under the covers, he positioned it palm down to facilitate an examination of his fingernails. He scrutinized each of them in turn and found three of the nails had abnormal white lines running directly across them. Each nail had a different number of abnormal lines, but they were all parallel to the cuticle.

A nervous roll settling in at the dome of his stomach, he walked across to the other side of the bed where he repeated the examination on the left hand. Two of fingernails had the same findings as the right.

"Glossitis and Mees lines," he whispered to himself, taking a gulp of air. Grabbing his phone, he hurried out of the room. After the fourth ring, he mumbled, "C'mon, Madison. For once, answer your phone."

She finally picked up on the next ring.

Before she could speak, he said, "What are you doing?"

"I was just about to do a quick check on Lori."

"Can that wait a few minutes?"

"I guess so. What the hell's going on, Jack? You sound excited... even for you."

"Meet me in John Winkler's room," he said with impatience.

"Right now?"

"Yes, Madison. Right now."

"Okay. I'll be there in a couple of minutes."

Jack walked slowly up and down in the corridor while he waited for her. The strange pacing was something almost subconscious he'd started doing many years ago when his mind would race. His confidence that he'd finally uncovered the first meaningful clue to unlocking the diagnosis was growing by the second. In an abundance of caution, he warned himself to tap on the brakes. He was critical of colleagues who shot from their hips, and he had every intention of not violating his own approach to diagnosing. There would be no victory dance until a lot more investigation was done to prove he had the right diagnosis. Madison's voice brought him out of his thoughts.

"What's going on, Jack?"

"Come with me. I want to show you something." Following him into the room, she said hi to Marietta, and then took up a position next to him at the head of the bed.

"Take a look at his tongue."

"Okay." Madison reached over to a box of examining gloves and slipped on a pair. She gently opened his mouth and examined his tongue. "It looks like he's got pretty significant glossitis. The inflammation definitely wasn't there yesterday, so it must be a new finding."

"I agree, but before you say anything else, take a look at his fingernails." She slipped her gloves off, tossed them into the trash, and put on a new pair. She began by picking up John's right hand. She studied it for a few seconds, stole a peek at Jack, and then examined the left.

"They look like Mees lines to me." Taking a couple of steps back, she lightly drummed her temple in thought. "There's no strain of encephalitis I'm aware of that causes either of those two findings, never mind both of them together. How about you?" He shook his head no. "There's something weird going on, buddy."

"I'd agree wholeheartedly."

"We only have ten minutes to get to Kristin's meeting. Let me think about this, and we'll talk about it as soon as it's over."

"I promised Anise we'd meet her in Nicole's room after the meeting and take her to dinner. We probably won't be able to talk until we get back to the hotel."

"That's only a few hours from now, Jack. C'mon, let's get going. I doubt it will escape anybody's attention if we walk in late."

"Give me another few seconds."

"Sure."

"I don't think the Marsh patients have viral encephalitis," he said with certainty.

"If you're saying we have an error in diagnosis, what do you believe is really going on?"

"I think they've suffered a toxic exposure."

"Excuse me?"

"I think they've been poisoned."

Part III

Chapter 32

Madison and Jack hurried to the fifth-floor conference room. She knew they only had a couple of minutes before the meeting started. It wasn't the time to begin a critical conversation she suspected would require all of her attention. On the other hand, and despite his impatience, she guessed Jack was actually a little relieved to have a few more hours to consider his theory in detail before sitting down with her. They both knew the feeling all too well of thinking they'd come across the first clue to making a tough diagnosis only to find out, as they drilled down on the possibility, that they were wrong.

When Jack and Madison entered the spacious conference room, most of the invited, including Aaron Steele, were already seated at the lacquered wood conference table. Jack and Madison were just about to join them when Erik walked over to greet them.

"I'm Erik Brickhill, the CEO of Marsh. It's a pleasure to finally meet you. I've heard nothing but wonderful things about you and your efforts to assist us with this problem."

"That's kind of you to say," Jack stated.

"Let's get together for lunch in the next few days. I'd like to get to know you both a little better."

"We look forward to it," Madison said.

"Great. I'll have my assistant reach out to you," he said, noting the last few stragglers entering the room. "I guess it's time to get this meeting rolling." He extended his hand. "It was a pleasure."

After he made himself comfortable in the chair next to Kristin, Erik held up a hand to quell the last few private conversations that were still going on.

"Let me begin by thanking everybody for attending this meeting on such short notice. I'd also like to extend my deep appreciation to all of you for your tireless efforts to help our colleagues. I'm going to depart from my incurable tendency to drone on and turn the meeting over to Dr. Hartzell, who I believe has some rather exciting news to share with us."

A surprised look passed between Jack and Madison.

"Did you know anything about this?" she whispered to him.

"No way. I was just about to ask you the same thing."

"Thank you, Erik," she said, sliding the few pages of notes she'd made a few inches closer to her. "As most of you know, our biggest obstacle in the care of the encephalitis patients has been our inability to identify the specific cause of the infection. Several days ago, our colleagues in the Surgeon General's office offered to help. They arranged for us to send various patient samples to the virology lab at the US Army Medical Research Institute at Fort Detrick. As I'm sure all of the physicians in the room are aware, this facility is considered to be as sophisticated and comprehensive a virology lab as any in the county." She stopped, picked up a crystal tumbler, and took a few sips of ice water. "Earlier today, I received a call from Dr. Alen Benedict, the director of the virology lab. He informed me they had successfully isolated an unusual strain of adenovirus in the samples of the spinal fluid we sent them."

Kristin's announcement stirred an immediate murmur in the room. After waiting for a few moments, she raised her hand, restoring silence.

Dr. Arch Britton was the first to speak. "You said an unusual type of adenovirus, Kristin. Can you be more specific?"

"According to Dr. Benedict, the strain was first recognized in New England about six months ago. It's close in appearance to

158

serotypes 3 and 7 but with some subtle differences. To his knowledge, no lab or hospital in the country has had much experience dealing with this particular strain."

"That's not encouraging to hear," Dr. Sue Novellino, the chief of infectious diseases, stated. "I've recently read about the strain Dr. Benedict's referring to. There's been some buzz about it across the country, but Kristin's quite correct, not too much is known about it, other than it seems pretty virulent."

"That probably also explains why it's not included in our routine viral panel testing and why all our results from the other labs have been negative," Elias Rutledge said.

"Did the folks at Fort Detrick have any theories or suggestions regarding treatment?" one of the other physicians in the task group asked.

"The only thing Dr. Benedict mentioned was that the clinicians he'd spoken to had tried cidofovir. Certain of the results were encouraging, while others were disappointing, which means I don't think we can draw any definitive conclusions from them. Other than that, I was unable to gather any information about possible effective treatments."

Arch retook the floor. "In spite of all the medications we've tried, the patients are all in a tailspin. Cidofovir's an FDA-approved drug, and we haven't tried it as yet. I don't know if the other physicians in the room would agree with me, but I feel that switching to it wouldn't be some wild shot in the dark." He looked up and down the table, opened his hands, and added, as if he were stating the obvious, "We have nothing to lose. I see no reason we shouldn't start it immediately."

Kristin looked over at Jack and Madison. "Your thoughts?"

"Based on the gravity of the situation, and assuming the patients have no contraindications to cidofovir, I'd tend to agree with making the change," Jack said. Madison agreed with a nod.

"Thank you," Kristin said. "Just to make sure we're all on the same page, are there any members of the physician group who are opposed to initiating cidofovir therapy as soon as possible?" Her question was answered by a guarded silence. She waited a few more seconds. When nobody at the table sought recognition, she took it to mean they were in agreement with Arch Britton's recommendation to start the new antiviral drug. "Since we all agree this is a necessary next step in our care of these patients, I'm going to ask Dr. Britton and Dr. Novellino to write the orders as soon as this meeting's over so we can begin the drug as soon as possible."

"We'll take care of it," Novellino told the group. "The first dose should be ready in a couple of hours. I'll check around the country to see if anybody's trialing a new antiviral drug that we might be able to get our hands on if cidofovir is ineffective."

"That's an excellent idea. Thank you."

"I assume we'll continue all of our other current therapeutic interventions," Elias stated.

"Of course," Kristin said.

The conversation about the new strain of adenovirus and possible treatments continued for the next thirty minutes. When there were no further questions or comments, Kristin asked, "Before we adjourn, do any of the physicians have anything else they'd like to share with the group?" There was no response. "In that case, I'd like to give Erik and Aaron the opportunity to provide us with their thoughts from the administrative side."

"Thank you, Kristin," Erik said. "While we understand this news in no way offers a guarantee that our coworkers will recover, the report is a breath of hope that we can find a way to cure this horrible illness and get our Marsh family members back to their lives. I hope this new information will be the beacon we've been praying for to light the path leading us to a cure for this dreaded illness. I know all of you have been burning the candle at both ends and have done everything in your power to help our colleagues. All we can do at this point is pray the new medication will eradicate the virus."

"Thank you, Erik," Kristin said, looking at Aaron to see if he'd like to say something as well. He gestured to the contrary. "If nobody has anything further, I think we can wrap things up."

The group came to their feet. Many milled around for a few minutes to further discuss the remarkable news that Kristin had just shared with them. Even though the certainty of a cure was hardly assured, the atmosphere in the room was one of unmistakable optimism.

Dr. Wilbur Davidson, a venerable internist who probably should have retired ten years ago, still came to work every day sporting a striped bowtie and ready to work. His memory wasn't what it once was, but his judgment and fund of knowledge were untouched by time. He had introduced himself to Jack and Madison soon after they had officially become involved.

"That was quite a meeting," he said, arching his bushy gray eyebrows. "I never expected to hear our microbiological culprit is a new strain of adenovirus. Boy, that came out of left field...and just in the nick of time. Pretty convenient, I'd say."

Jack said, "Sometimes a little good fortune comes your way when you least expect it."

"Truer words were never said, Jack." His eyes narrowed. "I saw John Winkler the day he was admitted. He was pretty sick."

"You won't get an argument from us on that one," Madison said, sensing Wilbur wasn't simply making idle chitchat.

"When his seizures were finally under control, he was actually semi-lucid for several hours. I saw him during that time." He cocked his head just slightly to the side. "We've all seen how scared people can get when they're seriously ill, but John was terrified...like there was something else going on." He shrugged his shoulders and then scrubbed his chin. "You're busy folks. I shouldn't waste your time with the eccentric clinical observations of an old curmudgeon. I'll have to be more careful to guard against doing that. It was nice seeing you." With the assistance of a derby-handled black cane, he walked away.

"What in the world was that all about?" Jack asked.

"I'm not sure, but he doesn't strike me as the type of individual who busies himself with idle prattle."

"What do you think it was that he purposely wasn't saying?"

"Maybe that things aren't always what they seem or appear and that we should put on our thinking caps," she answered with concern registered in her voice.

"For somebody who just received great news, Kristin wasn't exactly doing backflips."

"Maybe you're just saying that because it flies in the face of your toxic exposure theory."

"Well, it certainly gives me reason to pause and reconsider my flash of genius. But I still feel like she's not as convinced about the accuracy of the adenovirus culture as she wanted everybody in the room to believe."

"Which puts you in her camp," Madison said with a casual grin. "You just love playing devil's advocate with me."

"Maybe, but if you're going to try to convince me you're sold on the fact that we now have an irrefutable diagnosis—you'd better pull up a chair, 'cause you're going to be here for a while."

"I'm not convinced of anything. One culture report is hardly the voice of God. Even the most prestigious labs in the world aren't immune from making mistakes. Labs are staffed by human beings, Jack—they make errors from time to time. I can't wait until tonight when we have our *what if they're wrong* talk," she said in no uncertain terms. "C'mon, Anise is waiting for us."

By this time, the remainder of the attendees were slowly filing out of the conference room.

Aaron approached Kristin. "Do you have a moment to talk?"

"Of course, Aaron."

"Great. I need a few minutes to return a call I got during the meeting, but I don't want you to slip away on me."

"I don't mind waiting. I have a call or two to make myself."

"Great. I'll meet you right here in about ten minutes."

As he walked away, she groaned inwardly. She had a lot of patient care issues on her mind that required her attention. Wasting even a few minutes on some silly political matter Aaron was sure to present her with was not something she had any interest in doing.

Chapter 33

The moment she stepped off the elevator, Madison spotted Anise standing right outside the entrance to the intermediate care unit. She reached behind her and blocked Jack from moving out of the car.

"What's going on?" he asked.

"Why don't you go back down to the lobby for about fifteen minutes?"

"Excuse me?"

"Anise is down the hall. Give us a few minutes—this may be a good time for me to speak with her."

Without saying a word, he smiled and took a step back. "Good luck."

Madison walked down the hall and waved as soon as she caught Anise's eye. "Hi. How are you doing?" Madison asked.

"Okay, I guess."

"You're talking to an expert on how hard it is to stay patient."

"I feel like I'm in some kind of weird limbo... It's almost like time is standing still. All I do is worry about Mom and wait to get any hint from Dad or the doctors how she's doing." She gazed past

Madison down the hall. "Have you seen Dad? I thought you guys were coming together."

"He'll be here in about ten or fifteen minutes," she responded, trying to figure out the best way to broach the topic of Anise's state of mind. She was still pondering how to accomplish that when Anise took care of the problem for her.

"For the past few days, I've wanted to ask you about how you dealt with all the stress and fears of having leukemia."

She smiled at Anise. "We have a few minutes right now. Let's sit down and chat."

"Are you sure? Because if it's something you'd rather not talk about…I promise, I'll understand."

"I'm happy to answer any questions you might have about how I handled the emotional side of my illness. I'm also happy to talk with you about anything related to your mom's condition."

"The main thing is…and I don't want to upset Dad by mentioning this to him, but I don't think he gives me any credit for understanding things." After a few breaths to collect herself, she continued. "I'm really scared Mom's not going to pull through, and even if she does, I'm terrified she'll never be the person she was before she got encephalitis. Dad's being so careful not to upset me that I don't think he's being totally up front with me. I understand he's trying to protect me, but I'm not a ten-year-old. I own a laptop, and I know how to research a topic, even medical ones."

"I think you're right about him wanting to keep you a little sheltered and optimistic. But I can tell you that neither of us is convinced your mom's not going to fully recover."

A doubtful expression came to her face. "She's gotten worse every day since this horrible sickness started. Instead of everybody simply telling me she could pull through, I'd like to know specifically what her chances are."

"I don't think anybody knows that for sure." Not wanting to share what she'd just learned at the meeting with Anise, she continued, "I'm not going to tiptoe around the truth. If we can't find a specific treatment for your mom's illness, the chances of losing her go way up."

Anise lifted her downcast gaze. "When you were your sickest, were you still aware enough to know what was going on?"

Madison was tight-lipped for a few seconds. All she could manage was, "Sometimes I was, and sometimes I wasn't. It depended on a lot of things. After a while, you don't care if you're aware of what's going on around you. All you care about is living another day."

"That's what I'm worried about. Everybody thinks Mom can't hear or understand us, but I'm not so sure. Sometimes I'm sure she knows exactly what's going on and that she's terrified."

"She's getting a lot of medications to sedate her. Some of them even have the effect of blocking her memory. Speaking as a doctor, I can't imagine she's aware of anything."

"What went through your mind during your worst days?" Anise inquired.

"All I remember is that it was a roller coaster of emotions. There were days when I was on the brink of just caving in, praying for anything that would bring things to an end one way or another. And then there were other times, times I tried everything I could think of to make a deal."

"What do you mean by make a deal?"

"I'd promise any divine creation I thought might listen that I'd do anything in return for being allowed to live. I was ready to promise to do anything that was asked of me for the rest of my life." Madison paused to rub her eyes before going on. "Then there were other days that, no matter how sick I was, I somehow convinced myself that my time hadn't come yet, and no matter how much I was suffering, I was going to live to see another day." A faint smile came to her face. "When you're fighting for your life, you can make yourself believe almost anything."

"I…I just can't understand how you did it," Anise said.

"Sometimes, neither can I. What's strange is, I don't consider myself a very religious person. But at the time, I guess it was just the right combination of faith and optimism mixed with a whole bunch of mind games." After a telling pause, she added, "If there's any advice I can give you, I'd tell you not to listen to a lot of percentages and predictions based on people's notions about your mom's condition. Every patient is different, and every doctor is too. Your dad and I have both seen patients sicker than your mom pull through. The other thing is that if you look too far down the road, it can distort things and put you on the wrong track. What I'm saying is, stop thinking about next week and stay focused on right now."

"Thanks, Madison," she said, giving her a hug.

"You're welcome. Any time you need to talk, just come and find me."

Anise felt a tap on her back. She opened her eyes to see her dad behind her.

"Good timing," Madison said with a bit of a giggle.

Jack said nothing at first, looking at them both and noticing their eyes were a little on the moist side. He considered ignoring it but dismissed the notion for reasons he wasn't sure of.

"Hi guys," he said as his eyes moved across their faces. "Did I miss something?"

"You didn't miss anything, Dad. Madison and I were just talking."

"Really? What were you two—"

"It was girl talk, Jack, so take the hint."

He raised his hands in capitulation. "Nobody ever said I needed to be hit with a sledgehammer to get the idea." He put his arm around Anise. "C'mon, Shortstuff, let's go see Mom."

Chapter 34

While she waited for Aaron, Kristin couldn't help but wonder what was on his mind. Twenty minutes after he'd stepped out into the hall, he returned and took the seat next to her.

"Let me begin by sharing with you that everybody who's a member of the C-suite thinks you've done an incredible job managing an extremely difficult problem."

"Thank you."

"Based on the meeting, we're obviously much more hopeful that the remaining ten of our Marsh family patients are going to pull through, and everything will soon return to normal."

Kristin found his optimism compelling but suspect, especially since there was no evidence that any treatment would be successful.

He continued, "All of us in leadership are keenly aware you have enormous clinical and administrative responsibilities outside this current encephalitis problem. We were therefore thinking it might be a good idea to put another physician in charge of the medical side of things. Obviously, you'd still be involved in the day-to-day care of the patients. But we're concerned the enormity of the problem is taking too much time away from your many other responsibilities as our chief health officer."

"I'm getting the feeling you've convinced yourself the report we received today puts an end to the encephalitis problem. Granted, it's an encouraging piece of news…but we're still light-years away from a cure."

"I think we all realize that, but it's still the most optimistic and encouraging piece of news we've received since this terrible problem began." He leaned back in his chair and after pausing briefly, he went on. "There's something else I want to talk to you about. We feel it would be a good idea for you to step down from leading this initiative."

"Pardon me," she said, seated there looking stunned.

"Our concern is that you have so many other responsibilities that require your attention that perhaps your plate is getting too full. After all, we have other highly qualified physicians who could take the reins at this point."

Her stomach hardened and after a long moment, she said, "I really question the wisdom of your timing, Aaron. Passing the baton at this time could turn out to be a serious mistake."

"Normally, I'd completely agree with you, but this is a very unusual situation that the executive committee wants me to carefully supervise. So ultimately this change is my call."

"I see," she said more calmly tone. "Since it appears that this is a done deal, who did you have in mind to replace me?"

"I think Dr. Rutledge would be an excellent choice."

Feeling as if he'd already put a knife in her back and was now rotating it, Kristin warned herself not to lose her grip on civility as he continued speaking.

"He's an excellent man and has been an important member of the physician task group."

"Elias is a fine physician, but he's not employed by Marsh Technologies. With all due respect, he works for Georgetown Infirmary, and I'm not sure putting him in charge of the Marsh patients wouldn't be some kind of conflict of interest."

"That's a legal issue with more than one solution. But since I'm an attorney, why don't you leave that to me?"

"I see. May I remind you that I'm the admitting physician of record for all these patients, Aaron."

"That's more of an administrative technicality than anything else, isn't it?"

"Not if you're the physician of record." She held up a hand. "As long as you're assuring me that I'll continue in my clinical role caring for my patients, I have nothing more to say."

"I can assure you with complete impunity that we want you to continue having a role in the medical treatment of these patients. I might also mention that, in addition to freeing up some of your time, we also feel it might be better to shift to a doctor with more experience dealing with the media."

"So that's was this is all about. I should've known."

"Elias has significantly more experience than you do in dealing with the press and TV."

It immediately struck her that Aaron had finally found something they could agree upon. It was no secret that Elias embraced being center stage and rarely missed a photo opportunity. "You're still the chief of Marsh's employee medical program, but Elias will be fully responsible for this particular initiative and will be reporting directly to me," he explained. "I'm aware you and Elias don't have the best working relationship, but I would of course expect you two to put those differences aside for the good of the patients and work together in a collegial and productive manner."

Cringing inwardly from being treated like a problematic child, Kristin said. "I wouldn't have it any other way."

"You're always welcome to take the matter to a higher court," he said with an egotistical grin. "My self-image can handle it, although from a practical standpoint, I don't think you'll get very far."

"I never forget my manners, Elias, and I've never found it necessary to trample on one of my colleague's heads when I disagreed with him or her."

"I happen to agree with you, but it's part of Marsh's culture to park your ego at the door and feel free to talk to anybody about anything. I can tell you I've given this matter a good deal of thought, and I feel this isolated change of leadership is the best way forward for our company. I know you're disappointed, but I hope in time you'll see the...wisdom of this change."

Every time Kristin was convinced she'd heard Aaron's most disingenuous explanation, he surprised her by topping himself.

"Since we just learned about the new strain of virus that's causing the encephalitis, I assume you haven't discussed the prospect of this change with Elias yet."

"As I mentioned, you needn't concern yourself with the small details of the transition. Just leave that to me. I'm sure everything will work out fine," he said, getting up from his seat.

"I'm sure it will."

Unable to bear another nanosecond of the humiliating experience, Kristin stood up and marched out of the conference room before Aaron reached the door.

Chapter 35

FIFTH DAY

Plagued by the events of yesterday, Kristin sat behind her desk wondering why she couldn't shake the uneasy feeling that the news from the viral laboratory at Fort Detrick had sealed the fate of the Marsh patients. Understanding her patient responsibilities came first, she somehow managed to move her unpleasant meeting with Aaron to a remote corner of her mind.

Despite the small amount of optimism Dr. Benedict had shared with her about cidofovir's possible effectiveness in treating the new strain of adenovirus, she was beyond skeptical the drug would help any of the patients. She'd be the first to admit his call had caught her off guard, but she was still miffed at herself for not being more inquisitive about his lab's findings. Perhaps if she'd pressed him harder, with more questions, he would have remembered more. She hoped her failure to do so wasn't the reason for his disappointingly sparse information.

It was eight-thirty when she took the last bite of the blueberry muffin she'd purchased on her way to work. She again considered calling Dr, Benedict but was concerned about the possibility of annoying him by asking him to repeat information he'd just given her the day before. She continued to grapple with the prospect until she resigned herself to the fact that there were worse things in the world than being a pest. Finally, after exhaling a determined breath, she placed the call to the laboratory at Fort Detrick.

"This is Dr. Hartzell calling. I'd like to speak with Dr. Alen Benedict, please."

"I'll be happy to connect you, Doctor."

"Special Pathology Lab, Corporal Short speaking."

"This is Dr. Hartzell calling from the Georgetown Infirmary. I'm trying to reach Dr. Benedict."

"I'm sorry, Dr. Hartzell. Dr. Benedict left last evening on an urgent field assignment."

Surprised, based on what he'd told her about his availability for the next few weeks, Kristin asked, "Do you know when he's expected to return?"

"I'm sorry, Doctor. I don't have that information."

"Would you know if there's any way I can contact him by phone or email?"

"My understanding is that he's not reachable."

With her frustration climbing, she asked, "Is there somebody covering for Dr. Benedict whom I might be able to speak with?"

"I'll connect you with Dr. Tay. She's in charge of the lab until he returns."

"Thank you."

Based on her conversation with Short, Kristin didn't hold out much hope that anybody would be available to take her call, but to her surprise, Dr. Tay promptly picked up.

"Dr. Tay. How may I help you?"

"My name's Kristin Hartzell. I'm an internist at the Georgetown Infirmary. Dr. Benedict called me yesterday regarding the results of blood and spinal fluid samples we'd sent him from two of our patients whom we're treating for encephalitis. I had some follow-up questions for him, but I just learned he's been deployed and can't be reached. Corporal Short suggested I speak with you."

"Of course. I'd be happy to help you if I'm able. What were the results of those cultures?"

"They were all positive for a new strain of adenovirus. Dr. Benedict mentioned it was similar to 3 and 7, but I don't believe he provided me with a specific designation for the strain."

"I wasn't aware we'd seen another case of the adenovirus strain. I'm surprised Alen didn't mention it to me or tell me that you might be calling."

"I decided to call back in hopes that he might have recalled some additional information about the new strain. Our patients aren't doing well, and in an effort to be as thorough as possible... well, I didn't want to leave any stones unturned."

"I completely understand, and as much as I'd like to help you, Dr. Benedict's our local expert on adenoviruses. I can't imagine, even if I knew about the results, I'd have much to add beyond what he's already told you."

"Would it be possible for you to check the date you received the samples and the results for me?" Kristin asked, with what little optimism she had fading quickly. "We don't have a written report as yet, and I just want to be absolutely certain there hasn't been a lab error or some other administrative problem."

"I'd be happy to have a look for you. I just need a minute to get into our system and I'll bring up the studies and double-check everything,"

"Thanks. Do you need any of the patient names?"

"Probably not. I should be able to bring it up by using Georgetown Infirmary as the initiating institution." After a minute or so went by, Tay said, "I'm sorry, Dr. Hartzell. For reasons I don't understand, it seems like we failed to enter the basic intake information in our data bank. This is very unusual. Hopefully I'll be able to find the records, but it may take me some time. I'll have to give you a call back, but it might not be until tomorrow."

"So you can't even confirm you received the samples?"

"I can't find the cases in the computer, but seeing as how you discussed the results with Alen yesterday, they must be in there somewhere. Maybe there was a technical problem overnight that caused them to go missing. I'll get our IT folks involved as soon as possible. Hopefully, by tomorrow I'll have more information on the samples you sent. I think I will take the names of the patients from you."

Kristin provided the information she requested and added, "Let me give you my cell phone number so you won't have any trouble tracking me down. Thank you, Dr. Tay. I look forward to hearing from you."

Overcome with a mixture of confusion and disappointment, Kristin stared absently at the montage of photographs she'd hung on her wall of her various trips to Southeast Asia. The first decision she reached was that she wasn't going to sit tight and wait for matters to unfold on their own. She needed to proactively move things to a different level. There were a few options that might accomplish that, but she settled on the one she believed would bring the best results most quickly.

She reached for her phone.

"Hi, Jack. By any chance, are you and Madison free?" She listened briefly. "Great, can you guys spare me a few minutes? I have something rather confidential I'd like to talk with you about." She listened for a minute and responded, "Fifteen minutes would be fine. How about my office?" she asked. "Great, I'll see you then."

Sitting back in her chair, Kristin felt grateful for the few minutes she had before they'd arrive. Nervously drumming her desk, she felt like a conflicted governor nervously facing the approaching top of the hour, struggling to decide whether she should order a stay of execution or not.

Chapter 36

The fifteen minutes seemed to vanish, leaving Kristin startled by the two quick knocks on her door. She moved out from behind her desk and opened it for Madison and Jack.

"Thanks for coming up." She pointed to the two blue oak-frame chairs that faced her desk.

"No problem," Jack said.

As soon as Kristin retook her seat, she wasted no time in getting to the crux of what was on her mind.

"I have a significant concern regarding the lab report we received from the Army's viral lab that I'd like to discuss with you." When she noted the odd look that simultaneously crossed Jack and Madison's faces, she stopped and changed directions. "Is there something you guys would like to say first?"

"Only that you must be reading our minds," Jack said. "Madison and I had a long, sobering talk last night regarding the same topic. We were just about to call you to arrange a meeting to share our concerns when you beat us to it."

"This is getting more interesting by the minute. Who's going first?"

"It's your meeting," Madison said. "Why don't you start?"

Kristin interlocked her fingers and set her hands on the desk. "It seems the members of the physicians in our task group are quite willing to accept the accuracy of the adenovirus culture result from the Army virology lab. I'd agree with them that it seems to tie every-thing up in a nice bow. But it's only one report, and I'm having trouble blindly accepting its accuracy. So, just to verify their find-ings, I decided to call Dr. Benedict this morning to see if I could get some additional information. I was informed he'd been urgently deployed to an unnamed location and couldn't be reached. I was referred to a Dr. Tay, who was covering for him. She was helpful but informed me she didn't know anything about us sending samples to them or the results. When she checked their data bank, she was unable to locate any records of the specimens we sent them. She apologized for the screw-up, said she'd have their IT department look into it, and promised to call me when they figured out what happened." Holding any further thoughts, Kristin stopped drum-ming, placed her palms flat down on the desk, and gazed at them.

"You almost sound like you think there's some conspiracy going on," Madison said. The comment turned Jack's head in surprise. Even if the possibility had crossed her mind, he wasn't sure mentioning it was well advised.

"I don't know what I think," Kristin responded. "Jack?"

"I think we'd all be well served to keep our eye on the ball and for now confine our concerns to the medical aspects of these cases." After a strained but brief silence, he went on. "Regarding the Army lab, you might hear form Dr. Tay today or tomorrow with the news she found the records. And maybe she'll have some updated infor-mation on Dr. Benedict's availability. The whole thing could turn out to be some kind of administrative mix-up,"

"All I can say is that I hope you're right," Kristin said, looking unconvinced. "So tell me about this conversation you two had last night."

"To begin with, we don't believe the patients are suffering from any form of encephalitis," Jack said flatly.

"Excuse me?" she asked, her eyes searching his. "Madison, you feel the same way?"

She nodded. "We're worried Dr. Benedict's lab made a mistake."

Kristin opened the top right drawer of her desk and removed a pad. Leaning forward, she plucked her fountain pen from its black platinum stand.

"I'm not sure what convinced you of that, but don't stop now. I can't wait to hear this."

"Before we explain, I'd like to mention one medically unrelated point," he said.

"Sure, go ahead."

"What we think we may have stumbled across places Madison and me in the middle of an unmapped minefield. We're here as invited guests to lend our medical opinions without stepping on anybody's toes, especially those belonging to the physicians on the task group. I'm not suggesting we make any patient care compromises, but I'd like to move forward without rocking the boat too much."

Kristin drew back slightly and looked over at Madison with a furrowed brow. "What do you think?"

Jack cringed as he anticipated her response. He doubted it would surprise him.

"I don't care much about political nuances and strategies. If it means helping our patients, I'm happy to step on anybody's toes that happen to get in the way."

"I tend to agree with Madison on this one, Jack."

Jack cleared his throat but retreated into silence.

"Please feel free to rock the hell out of the boat, if that's what it takes. If there aren't enough trained therapists to go around to accommodate those with wounded egos, too bad. I'll take care of any unwanted political fallout."

Jack nodded and did his best to remain plain-faced, but he couldn't fight off the impression he was sitting in the very office where diplomacy came to die. Kristin rubbed her hands together with enthusiastic anticipation.

"Now, let's hear what you two have to say about our patients not having encephalitis."

Madison took the lead. "Just to review some of the stranger aspects of the cases before we get into some new areas: We all know that the great majority of viral encephalitis patients have a rise in their spinal fluid white blood cell count and protein level. And many of them have an abnormal brain MRI." She paused and held up her index finger. "None of the Marsh patients have any of these findings. In fact, the only abnormal finding is a low cholesterol level in almost all the patients. At first, we didn't know why, but we think we have an idea now."

Jack said, "There's one question that remains unanswered: transmission. If we're dealing with an adenovirus infection, we'd all agree that person-to-person transmission would be accounting for it. But adenovirus is transmitted like other airborne viruses, so it's hard to imagine how that happened when none of our patients experienced significant coughing, sneezing, runny nose, or any other infectious respiratory symptoms. It's also hard to point to an adenovirus as the culprit when only eleven people out of the thousand or so who work in the building were infected."

"Nobody can argue with that logic, Jack, and it's a question most of the task group doctors have been asking themselves since yesterday's meeting. Unfortunately, at least for now, it's nothing more than an interesting oddity whose answer might not turn out to be clinically important." She looked at them askance. "That being said, I suspect you have more to share with me."

With a nod from Madison, Jack continued, "I was making rounds on John Winkler yesterday and noticed he had fairly pronounced glossitis. I hadn't noted it before in him or any of the other patients, but when I went back and reexamined them, I found three others who also had an enlarged, inflamed tongue. I'm not aware of any form of viral encephalitis that causes glossitis." Jack held his next thought, setting his eyes on Kristin to see if she might have a question. When she didn't, he continued. "The presence of glossitis got me thinking and eventually prompted me to go back and examine John's fingernails."

"His fingernails?"

"That's right. And there's no question he has Mees lines on both hands."

"Are you absolutely sure?"

"The finding's undeniable."

"I'm a little rusty, but as I recall, Mees lines are usually found in patients with renal failure and certain malignancies."

"But never in encephalitis," Madison pointed out. She could see from the expression on Kristin's face that she was becoming more intrigued with the conversation.

"What else have you come across?" she asked, as she jotted down a couple of lines of notes.

"I've been with Anise a few times when she's visited Nicole," Madison said. "She generally sits right next to her at the head of the bed and lightly brushes her hair as she speaks to her. I didn't think much of it at first, but I remembered last night, when Jack and I were talking, that I saw Anise removing a few clumps of hair from the brush and tossing them in the trash." Kristin looked up from the pad. "So you're adding alopecia to the list of new findings."

"Yes, and as is the case with glossitis, hair loss has no association with viral encephalitis. Nicole's hair loss got me thinking about other possible findings we may have missed because we were so focused on encephalitis. That's when I remembered something Lori Somersby's wife, Gretchen, mentioned to me the first time I saw her. It was when you and Jack went to that meeting with Aaron Steele. Very early on in her illness, Lori was having trouble distinguishing colors. Gretchen told me she has no history of any type of color blindness. Then I remembered one of the other patients' spouses giving me a similar history, but I mistakenly wrote it off to double vision." She paused temporarily. "I decided to call Gretchen last night while she was still in the hospital. I asked her to brush Lori's hair to see if she noticed any excessive clumps of hair. She told me she didn't have to because she'd begun noticing it three days ago."

"But she didn't say anything?" Kristin asked.

"She told me she just assumed it was part of the illness or a side effect of one of the drugs Lori's on." Madison watched as Kristin pushed her palms together and rested her chin on her fingertips.

"So we have glossitis, Mees lines, color blindness, and hair loss," Kristin stated, regarding them through searching eyes. "Interesting group of signs and symptoms, which I assume led you to a lightbulb moment you're about to share with me."

"Mees lines can be associated with thallium and arsenic poisoning," Jack said.

"And temporary color blindness has been reported with mercury poisoning, and zinc toxicity can cause an abnormally low cholesterol," Madison informed her.

Appearing deep in thought, Kristin slowly came to her feet and moved around to the front of her desk where she stood directly in front of Madison and Jack.

"You mentioned arsenic, zinc, mercury, and thallium," Kristin said distinctly." Are you suggesting that the ten Marsh employees who are now hospitalized in our IMCU were all the victims of some type of *heavy metal poisoning?*"

Chapter 37

Kristin went silent while she walked over to a small refrigerator and removed a bottle of water.

"Can I get you guys something to drink?"

"I'll take a water," Madison said, while Jack politely refused by holding up his hand. She removed a second bottle, handed it to Madison, and retook her seat behind her desk.

"It's been a couple of decades since I read anything on heavy metal poisoning, so bear with me and fill in the blanks."

"Sure," Jack said.

"As I recall, most of the heavy metals are naturally occurring in our environment. I think the number of toxic ones varies among the experts, but if my memory serves me correctly, there are at least a couple dozen. I'd add chromium and lead to the ones you've already enumerated. But isn't it true that patients suffering from heavy metal toxicity tend to work in specific jobs in manufacturing and mining where the risks are well known? Their pathogenesis results from their ability to bind and accumulate in specific organs, which causes significant damage to them." Krisitin's gaze fell on both of them at the same time. "Is that about it in a nutshell?"

"I'd say the things you've mentioned are some of the key characteristics of heavy metal toxicity," Jack answered.

"Not to splash mud on your galoshes, but Marsh Technologies' corporate headquarters is an immaculately maintained office environment that is inspected and scrutinized for workplace safety several times a year."

"Right now, it's just a theory," Madison said. "We wouldn't begin to presume we have all the answers."

"I'm sure you're both aware that we did a toxicology workup on all the Marsh patients, which included all manner of toxins and poisons…not just heavy metals…that came back totally negative."

Jack said, "We understand that, but if you focus on the heavy metal studies we ran, it was a pretty basic workup."

"As I recall, most victims of heavy metal poisoning are affected by only one of them, and each of those metals has its own very specific cluster of symptoms and severity. Going back to the symptoms you mentioned—they seem to have come from three or four different heavy metals. How would that be possible?"

"Madison and I talked about that at length. We feel it's possible we could be dealing with some new heavy metal toxin that's never been seen before or possibly one that's a derivative or an altered form of one of the known heavy metals. If we're right about that, it would probably explain why the toxicology workup was negative."

Kristin turned her eyes toward the ceiling. "You're getting a little weird on me, guys. This theory's farther out there than the Milky Way." She looked back at them. "Tell me again how the Mees lines play into all this?"

"Mees lines can be seen with thallium, lead, and arsenic toxicity," Jack stated.

"Thallium? Wasn't that what they used in the manufacture of insecticides decades ago? But when they found out how toxic it was, the government banned its use." She raised her index finger and wagged it with the precision of a metronome. "Look, I appreciate you bringing this to me, but encephalitis and heavy metal poisoning seem pretty far apart to me. It's hard to imagine we could confuse one with the other."

"Actually," Jack began in his calmest tone of voice. "Many of the heavy metal exposures include an extensive number of neurologic symptoms that closely mimic encephalitis. The medical literature is full of case reports addressing all kinds of errors in diagnosis in patients who turned out to have heavy metal toxicity."

"I'm certainly not in a position to cast doubts in your direction on the topic of elusive diagnoses." She stopped long enough to reach into her center drawer, pull out a bottle of chewable Tylenol, and pop a couple into her mouth. "Correct me if I'm wrong, but I'm getting the distinct feeling you believe there's enough here to officially pursue the possibility we've made a mistake in our diagnosis and should turn our attention to proving our patients haven't been the victims of heavy metal poisoning."

"You're not wrong," Madison stated flatly.

"Which would mean our first stop would be taking this...this alternative diagnosis to the physician task group."

"That would seem to make the most sense," Jack said. "Or we could spend a little more time digging deeper into the possibility to strengthen our case before we pitch them."

"I don't think we have a little more time to spend," Kristin said, absent any hesitation. "How would you start?"

"We'd need to do a lot more research, and we need to find the most sophisticated labs in the country that are focused on heavy metal detection and research. Hopefully, that should lead us to a few experts in the field whose minds we can pick."

"The question is, how do we minimize any push-back we get from the other physicians?" Madison asked.

"Off the top of my head, I can think of two things," Kristin said. "We emphasize the imperative of being absolutely certain we haven't overlooked an alternative diagnosis, specifically a toxic exposure. We can then point out that our current therapy doesn't have to be changed as we look into the possibility of a heavy metal exposure."

"That seems to make sense," Jack said.

"There's one other alternative, although I can't say it would be my first choice," Kristin said. "We could simply say nothing and start our own low-key diagnostic evaluation."

Madison grinned and said, tongue in cheek, "My aunt once told me that sometimes it's better to ask for forgiveness afterward than permission before."

"I think that only works if you're a kid," Jack said.

"Well, it won't be you two who'll get summoned hauled into some bigwig's office to answer a lot of prickly questions on the ethical treatment of one's colleagues."

"Let's just play it straight," Jack suggested. "Keeping things above-board is the safest way to go."

"That settles it. Full and honest disclosure it is," Kristin said. "So the next question is timing. We have our daily meeting with the group today. Do we drop the bomb then or give ourselves another day or two to airbrush our pitch?"

"At the risk of being redundant, we don't have time for any slow-moving strategies or dilly-dallying," Madison said. "I vote for a meeting today. Jack, your thoughts?"

"I'm all in for that option."

"Okay. That's it, then," Kristin said. "One thing—this is your plank to walk. I'll back you all the way, but I'm leaving the presentation to you two."

After a brief silence, they all came to their feet, and Kristin escorted them out of her office. As they were strolling down the hall toward the elevators, she mentioned, "Assuming we don't hit a brick wall at the meeting, I have a suggestion where we might want to start."

"We're all ears," Madison said.

"I don't usually advocate this in the practice of medicine, but it's crunch time and we need a shortcut. Living in the area, we have a physician by the name of Ralph Pike who's probably one of the most experienced toxicologists in the country. I've called him over the years a few times to get his input on a case. I wouldn't exactly call us friends, but I think I know him well enough to request a face-to-face meeting. It may be wishful thinking, but I think he'll agree."

"Where does he work?"

"The University of Maryland Medical Center, but he's semi-retired now."

Madison spoke right up. "We're not in a position to turn down any credible help. I think meeting with him is a great idea."

"Okay," Kristin said. "I'll give it my best shot and let you know."

Chapter 38

After the task group meeting, Jack and Madison walked out of the room with Kristin.

"You guys gave a great presentation," Kristin said.

"I expected more discussion," he stated. "I'm not really sure how well our pitch was received.

"I could've gone a lot worse. I expected Elias to lead a thundering opposition charge, but he was uncharacteristically subdued. My best guess is that we may be in a honeymoon period. Now that he's in charge, he may have intentionally kept a low profile to give himself the time he needed to make a few well-placed phone calls. Bottom line—I doubt we've heard the last from him on this matter."

Madison said, "I think we did okay for an opening salvo. My impression was that most of the group was skeptical about investigating a possible toxic exposure but had no serious objections to doing it. Maybe that's the most we can ask for at this point. At this point, we don't need their resounding support. For now, I'll settle for a simple go-ahead nod."

"I've been working with these folks for a long time. I've learned that sometimes it can be hard to read them. They can be a little squirrelly and unpredictable, especially after somebody persuasive gets their ear. But being the eternal optimist that I am, I called Dr. Pike to set up a meeting, and he agreed."

"Great," Madison said. "When is it?"

Kristin glanced at her watch. "In about three hours."

"Really?"

"He invited us to come to his house today at four."

"We certainly can't be accused of allowing any grass to grow under our feet," Jack said.

"Walk with me," Kristin said. "Dr. Pike's going out of town tomorrow, which isn't a problem except for the fact that I have a mandatory meeting in a few hours with Marsh's C-suite, which means you two will be on your own for the meeting."

"We'll be okay," Madison assured her. "We can brief you as soon as we get back."

They walked with her across the skybridge that led to the educational center.

"Did I mention that Dr. Pike recently celebrated his ninety-eighth birthday? To say he's of sound mind and body would be an enormous understatement. I think you'll find him amazingly sharp. Good luck. I can't wait to hear all about it," she said, disappearing into the educational center.

"Things are certainly getting interesting," Madison said. "I'm sorry. I should have asked sooner, but how's Nicole doing?"

"She's a little worse. Arch was in her room when I got there. Neither of us thinks the antiviral drugs are doing her or any of the other patients much good. The one piece of encouraging news is that her pulmonary function is improving. He thinks they may be able to get her off the vent in a couple of days. Unfortunately, her kidney and neurologic function are worse. Arch wants her to have another MRI of her brain later today. I didn't say anything, but I'm not sure what that's going to add at this point."

"I'm so sorry, Jack. What about Anise? Have you spoken to her today?"

"Not yet. Last night she told me she'd be here sometime this afternoon. She's obviously still depressed but hanging on," he said, his voice trailing into a dismayed tone. "On the positive side, I think the talk you had with her helped."

Madison studied Jack's stooped posture and the drained look that had settled on his face. She was disappointed in herself for not being more aware of his advancing level of stress. Between Nicole's struggle for life and the devastating impact it was having on Anise, his stress level was becoming toxic. His lingering anxiety related to her fight with leukemia and the extreme professional demands of consulting on difficult cases only made matters worse. She knew him well enough to realize he'd do everything in his power to hide the toll the pressure was leveling on him. Better than some, she understood that there was just so much any one person was capable of giving. She was suddenly consumed with fear that Jack was getting dangerously close to the point where he'd given all he was capable of.

Chapter 39

After a ride during which they somehow managed to escape the usual Washington traffic, Madison and Jack pulled up in front of the home of Dr. Ralph Pike, a two-story Williamsburg Revival in Baltimore's quaint Federal Hill neighborhood. He'd lived there for the past fifty-one years, never having given serious thought to moving. Embracing his father's teachings on the importance of punctuality, Jack arrived fifteen minutes early for their meeting.

"Maybe we should talk about the obvious question he's going to ask before going in," Madison said.

"What do you mean?"

"C'mon, Jack. He's going to ask if we think the toxic exposure was an act of God or somebody's intentional undertaking."

"Let's not get ahead of ourselves. We don't even know if Dr. Pike will agree with us that we're dealing with some type of poisoning."

"Just for the sake of argument, let's say he does."

"I say we play it by ear."

"Great answer, Jack."

He grinned. "C'mon, let's go meet the professor."

They exited the van and walked up the bluestone-paved driveway. Jack banged the brass doorknocker a couple of times, and in short order, a gaunt, bald-headed man wearing baggy black cargo jeans and a Scotch plaid flannel shirt opened the door. His facial skin was thin and weathered. A nest of fragile blood vessels, some ruptured, stretched down from beneath his eyes to reach the lower border of his cheekbones.

"You must be Drs. Wyatt and Shaw. Please come in," he said with a warm smile and a gravelly voice.

"Thank you, Dr. Pike. It's a pleasure to meet you," Madison said. "We can't thank you enough for agreeing to speak with us."

"I was honored to receive Kristin's call. Come, we can sit in my library and chat." He escorted them down the center hall. Jack was surprised to see how spry he was, walking sturdily, without the assistance of even a cane.

Having officially retired as a full professor of forensic pathology with both an MD and a PhD in toxicology, Pike had been granted emeritus status and still sporadically attended conferences and consulted at the medical school. A little to his surprise, he didn't miss his research and clinical activities in the slightest, but he did pine for his many colleagues and the hundreds of medical students and residents whom he'd inspired and instructed during his tenure on the faculty of the medical school. By the time he retired, he was regarded as an international authority on a wide array of toxic exposures.

After Jack and Madison were seated on the lumpy upholstered couch, Pike slid in behind his desk and settled into his leather manager's chair. The house was several degrees warmer than Jack preferred, and the scent of cooked fish pervaded the air. To Jack's surprise, there were no framed academic diplomas, awards, or certificates of achievement hanging on the walls.

"I was sorry to hear that Kristin couldn't make our meeting."

"She was very disappointed as well. I know she was quite anxious to discuss the Marsh patients with you," Jack said.

"Forgive me. I'm forgetting my manners. Can I offer either of you something to drink?"

"I think we're both fine," Madison answered.

"Good. The walk to the kitchen seems to get tougher by the day," he said with a disheartened grin. "So let's get down to business," he added, scrubbing his hands together. "Based on what Kristin told me, you're worried your current diagnosis of encephalitis may be incorrect. Is that about the gist of things?" Both Jack and Madison nodded. He was blunt, Jack would grant him that. "If it's not a virus, and you're sitting in a toxicologist's den, I'm forced to conclude you're concerned you may be dealing with a toxic exposure."

"That's precisely what we're worried about."

"Kristin told me your toxicology workup was both thorough and negative. I also understand you have a positive adenovirus culture from a highly reputable viral laboratory." He removed his horn-rimmed glasses, reached for a microfiber cloth, and took a few moments to polish the lenses. As he was refolding the cloth and placing it back in his desk drawer, he inquired, "Tell me, what sounded the alarm that your presumptive diagnosis was wrong?"

"It might help if we take you through the illness right from day one to where we stand today," Jack suggested.

"By all means."

Jack took a full twenty minutes to give Dr. Pike a comprehensive review of the Marsh patients' battles against encephalitis. With his chin resting on the back of his hand, Pike listened attentively, only interrupting once to request a clarification of something Jack said.

"The most common way people become exposed to a toxin is by ingestion, inhalation, or direct contact through the skin. Assuming you two are correct, what's your theory as to how the Marsh employes were exposed?"

"Unfortunately, at this point, we don't have the first clue," Madison answered.

"Well, based on the information you've given me, I'd have to agree with you that a toxic exposure is possible. But, as I'm sure you're aware, there are literally thousands of toxins out there, which begs my next question: Have you narrowed down the possibilities?"

Suspecting he knew the answer to his own question, Jack responded, "Based on the symptom complex and the way the illness has progressed, we're concerned we may be dealing with a heavy metal poisoning."

"Really? That's interesting, Jack. Do you have a particular one in mind?"

"Well, since the symptoms don't specifically fit one of the known heavy metal toxicities, and we don't have a clear history of an exposure, we can't say with certainty which one it might be."

"I'm sure you're aware that the commercial assays readily available for heavy metal analysis are pretty comprehensive and accurate."

"We are," Madison said.

Leaning forward, he set his elbows on his desk. "Heavy metals are certainly a fascinating topic within the field of toxicology. It has always fascinated me how, on the one hand, some can be poisonous in high doses, but on the other hand be essential for human survival in trace amounts. The unfortunate truth is that a lot of the problems with these metals have been caused by man's meddling with the environment and his foray into unsafe manufacturing practices. It's that type of negligent behavior that has poisoned way too many unsuspecting adults and innocent kids." He thumbed his ear briefly before going on. "If you don't mind, I'd like to pose a question of my own."

"Of course," they said at the same time.

"Assuming your patients have been the victims of a toxic heavy metal, do you think it was by accidental means, or did somebody have a hand in this?"

Madison cleared her throat as a *you should have listened* look came to rest on her face.

"As consultants on these cases, we feel it would be best if we stayed focused on the medical aspects of the illness. At this point, we're not even sure we're dealing with a toxic exposure."

Pike allowed his head to bob from one side to the other. "That was a safe answer, Jack. But suppose I complained to you that your response was probably a tad on the evasive side?"

Being impressed, and slightly amused, by Dr. Pike's mental

agility and no-nonsense persona, Jack wasn't offended by his inquiry.

Doing her best to conceal a grin, Madison said, "That's a pretty direct question."

"Those are the only kind I pose, young lady," he said with a faint smile. "But allow me to expand on it for a moment with an example of what I'm trying to point out. A physician treating a traumatized child is responsible not only for attending to the injuries but also for making a judgment as to whether those injuries occurred in a non-accidental manner. Do you agree?"

"I do."

"Good. Because I think your problem in Georgetown might turn out to be a similar situation."

Jack reentered the conversation. "I understand that arsenic and thallium and some of the other heavy metals have been used for criminal purposes. But, irrespective of how these individuals contracted the disease, our focus has to be on finding a cure. I'm not saying the circumstances surrounding the illness aren't important or should be ignored—I'm saying we should work our side of the street and let the authorities work theirs."

"Dare to dream, my boy. I only pray you'll be able to separate the two." Pike shifted his gaze to his treasured grandmother clock with its ornate moondial. "If you'll please excuse me for a few minutes, I have two cats I must attend to. They become unmanageable if I don't feed them at exactly the same time every afternoon."

"Of course," Madison said, successfully withholding a grin.

"Please be patient. I'm afraid I can't complete my household chores as quickly as I once could." He came to his feet, fixing his eyes on them both. "When I return, would you two be interested in hearing some interesting historical facts about dubious heavy metal research that might shed some light on your diagnostic predicament?"

"I'm sure we would," Jack told him with no hesitation.

He smiled, nodded his head once, and strolled out of the room, leaving Jack and Madison sitting there looking more than a little intrigued.

Chapter 40

Following her usual route down Virginia Avenue toward the Watergate Office Complex, Regan jogged with her shoulders hunched against a wet gusty tailwind that pinched at the nape of her neck. When she'd left her condominium forty-five minutes earlier, it was a temperate afternoon with a shallow ceiling of slow-moving cumulous clouds. Being familiar with how schizophrenic the DC weather could be in the late fall, she was hardly surprised by the abrupt change in conditions.

Five minutes later, her eyes fell on the Watergate office buildings, which marked the halfway point of her run and the landmark she used as her turnaround point. Looking at the eleven-story metal and concrete superstructure always reminded her of the centerpiece role it had played in one of the more notorious events in American history.

With situational awareness ever present in her mind, she took ten seconds to scan her surroundings. The moment she finished, she received a text reminding her to consider the vacation opportunities showcased by an upscale Jamaican resort she'd visited a few years ago. Recognizing it as this month's red text alert, she stopped instantly and called a ride-share company.

Fifteen minutes later, she stood in the living room of her condo looking at the District Wharf. She reached for her phone and made the call to the only number she had programmed into it.

"What took you so long?"

"I was out for a jog. I'd rather have some privacy when we talk, so I came home before I called."

Regan had only met Sol once. It was at the time she was completing her last two months in the Marine Corp. She'd accepted the three-hour interview request at the behest of her commanding officer. Since that day, all their communications were carried out by phone.

"Things are starting to get pretty interesting," he said.

"I guess that depends on your definition of interesting."

"It seems that Drs. Wyatt and Shaw have formed an unholy trinity with Kristin Hartzell."

"That's one way of putting it."

"Is there any other way?" he asked.

"Sometimes things are simply what they appear. Maybe they're just being conscientious doctors."

"I guess it's possible, but there are those of us who aren't willing to take that chance."

While she listened, Regan gently kicked a multi-colored soccer ball back and forth between her feet. It was the same one from high school that she'd made sure to bring with her to every place she'd ever lived.

"It seems like the efforts to diminish Dr. Hartzell's authority haven't done much to take the edge off her enthusiasm. It's also becoming pretty clear that the three of them are more than a tad skeptical that the Marsh patients are suffering from viral encephalitis."

"What convinced you of that?"

"Well, because even as we speak, Doctors Shaw and Wyatt are meeting with Dr. Ralph Pike, who just happens to be a renowned toxicologist," he informed her. "Try to remember that those who engaged us did so to ensure things like that wouldn't happen. Just because the government isn't directly involved doesn't mean they're not still quite intent on avoiding an embarrassing situation."

"I think things bear watching, but I'm not sure we need to go into panic mode."

"From what you're saying, I assume you're unaware of what happened at the doctors' group meeting earlier today."

"I'm in my own trench Sol, which means I don't get invited to the doctors' meetings. That's why I rely on you to keep me briefed on the most recent developments in a timely manner."

"The main topic of conversation was introduced by Dr. Hartzell but presented with her strong support to the group by our Ohio guest physicians. Apparently, they broached the possibility that the Marsh patients were exposed to a toxic chemical. The people you and I answer to got wind of it and contacted me with their collective underwear in a knot."

"Is anybody suggesting that this alleged poisoning was intentional?" Regan asked.

"No such suggestion was made…at least not yet. Dr. Wyatt made most of the presentation and never hinted that it could have been intentional. The prevailing opinion at the end of the meeting was that, if a toxic exposure did occur, it must have been an unfortunate environmental accident. We'd obviously like to see it stay that way."

Regan stopped tapping the soccer ball, sat down on her camelback love seat, and slid forward to the edge.

"I'll admit that Dr. Hartzell isn't exactly staying in her lane, but since she works for Marsh, wouldn't the smart move be to reassign her somewhere else."

"In the first place, Regan, we don't speak for Marsh, and in the second, I seriously doubt if they decided to do that, she'd go quietly into the night. As I mentioned, Marsh has already made some changes in her responsibilities that haven't done much to dampen her determination. Even if such a change could be made, that would still leave Drs. Wyatt and Shaw in play."

"They're invited consultants. Marsh can uninvite them any time they want."

"Get rid of them without good reason? The last thing C-suite wants is a firestorm of attention from within the organization, the families, or the media. Need I remind you that Jack Wyatt and Madison Shaw are pretty well known and highly respected—some folks might even call them national heroes. So I wouldn't hold my breath if you're waiting for Marsh to make a move like that."

If Regan had learned anything about Sol during their long relationship, it was that he was masterful at not displaying any emotion by the tone in his voice. That talent made it difficult for her to know what was really occupying the front of his mind and just how much importance he was placing on it.

"Cut to the chase, Sol. I'm always happy to offer an opinion, but I'm more on the execution side of the things we do. Where do you want me to go with this?"

"You have carte blanche to deal with this problem. Find a way to dissuade the three of them from pursuing the idea that the patients could be the victims of an any type of toxic exposure. Their job is to stay focused on encephalitis as the unequivocal diagnosis and the overwhelming likelihood that it will be fatal in all cases."

"You're aware that one of the patients is Wyatt's ex-wife."

"I am," he answered. "I'm also aware he has a daughter who loves her mother very much."

"It doesn't look like you're giving me much wiggle room here."

"You don't need any wiggle room, Regan— you just need to do your job. From where I'm sitting, it seems you have several options available to you. Need I remind you that in our business patriotism and efficiency trump everything."

"I'm well aware of that." She was about to remind Sol that she had an abiding love of her country and didn't need him or anybody else to instruct her on how to salute the flag. But Regan remembered something her father once told her: The boss wasn't always right but the boss was always the boss. Understanding his advice and the crucial importance of restraint, she said nothing further.

Sol went on, "If you were looking for a profession with a guaranteed voice and a choice in everything, you should've become a politician. A lot of what we do involves persuasion through education. I'm suggesting you educate these doctors as to the possible consequences of attempted heroic behavior on their part. If you need some help doing that, I'll make sure you have the usual assets at your disposal."

Sol's instructions were clear, although she was a little miffed by his delay in sharing key information with her. She wasn't a mind reader, but dwelling on her annoyance at his communication skills wasn't going to get her closer to where she needed to be.

Regan had never been able to think well on an empty stomach, which prompted her to get up and head into the kitchen to rummage around for something to eat. While she polished off the remainder of last night's baked ziti, she pondered her current situation. She'd have to work out the details, but she was supremely confident she'd find a way to make the annoying trinity understand their encroachment into areas that didn't concern them wouldn't go unnoticed or be tolerated.

Chapter 41

"What do you two know about the Horn Island Testing Center?" Pike inquired. He raised his index finger and lightly flicked the corner of his mouth.

Madison and Jack traded baffled looks. "I'm afraid, nothing," she said.

"During World War II, the government established a biological weapons testing site on a small island off the coast of Mississippi. The facility was an extension of the main research center at Fort Detrick. Initially, the experiments involved the use of insects as possible bioweapons in anticipation of the battles that were destined to take place in the Pacific. The center also looked at weaponizing botulin and ricin in the form of a bomb. Ultimately, the results were disappointing, the research records were sealed, and the projects were abandoned—except for one notable exception, which remained active from the end of the war to well into 1946. The work was highly classified and focused in part on exploring the feasibility of utilizing heavy metals as a potential weapon."

"Do you know which heavy metals were used?" Madison asked.

"Chromium, cadmium, mercury, and lead, among others. It's believed some of the experiments addressed the possibility of altering a heavy metal or combining them to create a potent contact poison."

"I'm not sure I understand," she said. "If there was no record of the work, how do you know so much about it?"

"Because I was stationed on Horn Island, Dr. Shaw. I was a senior lab technician at Fort Detrick, where most of the research on biological warfare was being done. But when the Army decided to open their facility on Horn Island, I was transferred there. When our commanding officer notified us the facility was to be closed, he ordered us to pack up all the records. A couple of days later, a truck showed up. We loaded it with every box we'd packed. Supposedly, they were being taken to a waiting Navy ship. There was no shortage of rumors about where the boxes were headed. The one that seemed most likely was that military intelligence was going to get all the material, but nobody knew for sure."

"As I recall, didn't the golden age of bioweapons take place in the 1960s?" Jack inquired.

"That's right, but Nixon eventually shut down the whole program. We could talk all day about what became of all that research, but it would be pure conjecture. Obviously, those I've spoken to over the years who were knowledgeable on the topic always pointed to various government agencies, especially the CIA. As the years went by, it became generally accepted that the information, by uncertain means, had also fallen into the hands of foreign government intelligence organizations and even criminal elements."

Pike stood up and walked in a slightly stooped posture over to a closet. He opened the door. The closet wasn't particularly large, but all the usable storage space was consumed by various-sized boxes and file folders. Pike had used a bold black marker to identify the contents of each box. Humming a catchy tune, he stood in front of the closet gazing up and down at its contents.

"There it is," he suddenly announced. "What do you say, Jack? How about helping an old curmudgeon get one of these boxes down?"

"Sure," he answered, getting up and making his way over to the closet.

Pike pointed as he spoke. "It's the little one there, on the left." Jack had no trouble reaching up, securing the box, and bringing it down. "Set it down there on my desk, please."

Madison joined them as Pike struggled with a wobbly hand to flip the lid off. Jack was just about to lend a hand when he decided to give him a few more seconds to avoid possibly denting his ego. A few moments later, Pike managed to pop the lid off. He wasted no time, immediately starting to flip through the manila file folders, persisting until he located the one he was after. His achievement was marked by a self-satisfied smile. He looked at it for another few moments before handing it to Madison.

"When I was stationed at Horn, three men I worked with were accidently exposed to a specific heavy metal they were trying to synthesize. Obviously, in those days the emphasis on safety and the techniques of assuring an accident-free research facility were a drop in the bucket compared to what they are today."

"What happened to them?" Madison asked.

"They all recovered, but it wasn't until after they'd been pretty damn sick for about a week."

"What was the nature of the illness?" Jack asked.

"Mostly a cluster of various neurologic symptoms."

"Did you transfer them off the island to a hospital?"

He chuckled. "Heavens no. We were at war, and our work was a top-secret operation. Horn had its own clinic. It was small, but it was staffed by a physician and two nurses."

"Did you eventually succeed in your experiments?" Madison asked him directly.

"No. But had we taken the work any further, or if some other group picked up where we left off...well, it's possible they could have pulled it off. The other thing you have to consider is that we have no idea how many similar research facilities existed in the world or for how long they continued operating. There was our facility at Fort Detrick, plus we suspected France, England, and Russia were also conducting similar research. The big question that remains is how much, if any, of this information fell into the wrong hands." Pike put his hand down on his desk to rest briefly. "Anyway, that file I gave you has my personal notes on the three men who were accidently poisoned on Horn Island. Feel free have a look at it."

"Are these documents still classified information?" Jack inquired.

"They're my personal notes. They were never classified."

"We'll be sure to have a careful look at these records and get them back to you as soon as we can," Madison said, shifting her gaze to Jack. "We've already taken up too much of your time. We should be going."

Pike took a few moments to replace the lid on the box and then waited while Jack replaced it in the closet.

"It was a pleasure speaking with you," he said, leading the way back to the entranceway. "I only hope I've been able to help you in some small way. I don't know if anything I've told you or something in my notes will help you in the care of your patients, but my reason for sharing my recollections and written accounts with you is to give you some idea of what was and is possible."

"Thank you, Dr. Pike," Jack said as they reached the foyer.

"Good luck with those patients. Please feel free to call me if you should have any more questions. And there's one other thing. Governments have some funny ideas of the best way to ensure and preserve their national security, especially if a high-ranking member or members have been embarrassed." Neither Jack nor Madison responded to his comment.

Madison was just about to walk out the door when she suddenly stopped and turned around.

"May I ask you one last question, Dr. Pike?"

"Of course. From that look on your face, I'm betting it's a doozy."

"You mentioned you had a couple of colleagues who had a particular interest in heavy metal exposures."

"That's correct. I do."

She clasped her hands together. "I was just wondering, if we were able to provide you with a few blood and spinal fluid samples, do you think they—or one even just one of them—might be willing to take a look at them and offer an opinion?"

"I think so. The person who comes to mind is Dr. Jenna Corsair. She's a longtime colleague of mine, astoundingly brilliant, and a very gracious person—probably just the type of individual you had in mind. I'll check with her today. If she's willing, I'll send you the address of her lab, and you can arrange to send the samples directly to her."

"Thank you so much."

Madison stole a peek at Jack to get a sense of his reaction to her request. Since he'd already averted his eyes and turned to the side, she wondered if she'd be hearing about her presumptive nature on the ride back to DC. They walked down the driveway and climbed into the van.

"He certainly made a point of sharing a lot of history with us," she said. "I don't know about you, but he stayed about three steps ahead of me the entire time we were there." Shaking her head slowly, she added, "If by some miracle I live to be his age, I hope I'm half as sharp as he is."

Chapter 42

After a leisurely dinner at an Asian restaurant, Jack and Madison walked the few blocks back to the Hay-Adams. They were crossing the lobby when a young lady wearing a plain blue-gray suit came up alongside them. Madison's initial thought was that she was part of the managerial staff.

"Excuse me," she said, discreetly removing her badge wallet and showing them her credentials. "I'm Special Agent Frankie Banks with the Federal Bureau of Investigation. I wonder if I might have a few minutes of your time?"

"What's this about?" Jack asked.

"Why don't we have a seat on the other side of the lobby, and I'll be happy to answer that question."

Banks was of average height, had a subdued smile, and tapered green eyes. She wore her light ash brown hair pulled straight back. Upon her graduation from Brown University's College of Law, she'd gone to work for the United States Attorney's Office for the District of Rhode Island. In her third year, she finally gave in to her life's dream to become a special agent with the FBI. It took her a full nine months to complete the rigorous application process to the Bureau, which included an eighteen-week course at the FBI

Academy in Quantico. Upon completion of the curriculum, she had proudly accepted a position as a special agent. That was five years ago almost to the day.

As soon as they were seated, Madison asked, "How can we help you, Special Agent?"

"I'm investigating the death of two Marsh Technologies employees that took place near Newport News, Virginia, a little over a year ago. I just have a few questions I'd like to ask you."

Madison frowned. "Did either of us know these individuals either professionally or personally?"

"I'm fairly certain you didn't. It's a fairly complex situation. All I can say is that the FBI doesn't make a habit of wasting citizens' and our agents' time speaking to people who have no hope of helping us."

"Does this have anything to do with the patients at Georgetown Infirmary?" he inquired.

"That's one of the possible connections I'm looking into."

"We'll be happy to answer your questions as long as they don't violate any ethical or legal guidelines," Madison hurried to make clear.

"I understand." Banks reached into her purse and removed a small spiral notebook and a black pen. "Obviously, I'm not a physician, but I am interested in learning what your impressions are of the encephalitis cases."

"I'm sorry," Jack said. "But are you able to tell us how you've gone from two unsolved murders in Virginia to our patients here in the Infirmary?"

"I understand your concerns, Dr. Wyatt, but I'm not asking you to disclose any specific patient information. I assure you, I'm familiar with HIPAA guidelines," she explained. Jack noticed her eyes continuing to scan the lobby area as she spoke. "As I just alluded to, the FBI wouldn't have an interest in this information if we didn't have good reason."

"Good reason can mean different things to different people," Jack said politely.

She flipped her notebook cover back and frowned. "Let me ask you this—looking at the patients as a group, are you expecting them to recover?"

"We have no way of predicting the eventual outcome for each patient," he answered.

"These individuals weren't together in an area where the types of mosquitos and ticks that transmit viral encephalitis are endemic. Have you ever seen an outbreak of encephalitis like this before?"

Madison answered, "I think both Dr. Wyatt and I would be comfortable saying this is a unique situation."

"Do you have a theory as to how they could have contracted the illness?" A passing but strained silence ensued. "You're not under oath, Doctors. These questions are routine."

Madison said, "We understand that but we're just trying to be sure that you're not getting into areas that could violate patient confidentiality."

Banks struck Jack as experienced when it came to interviewing a reluctant individual. While he appreciated her attempts to assure them her questions were purely routine, he wasn't as convinced as he suspected she would like him to be. It seemed clear that Special Agent Banks was exploring the possibility that the Marsh patients hadn't contracted this terrible disease by some random act of God. He looked to Madison for guidance. With her approving nod, he decided to be a little more forthcoming. "If we didn't have a positive culture confirming that an adenovirus is responsible for the illness, we could postulate other possibilities."

"Other possibilities? That's interesting. Tell me about that, Dr. Wyatt."

"As of right now, we have a culture that confirms the patients are suffering from a viral encephalitis. Any other diagnosis would be speculative."

"About that culture—do you have any reason to suspect the result they're reporting could be a laboratory error?"

"Lab errors occur, but as of right now, we have no reason to suspect there's been a mistake," Madison said.

"If, in the days to come, you found out there had been an error of some type, would you be surprised?"

"Special Agent," Madison asked directly, "why don't you just ask us if we believe the Marsh patients were the victims of an intentional act to harm them?"

"Could they have been, Dr. Shaw?"

"We're not in a position, from a medical standpoint, to rule out anything, but we'd like to make it clear something like that would be way outside our purview as medical consultants."

"Have any of the patients' families or coworkers said anything that has shed greater light on the illness?"

"We continue to gather information from several sources to help us in the care of these patients. Beyond that, I'm afraid we can't be any more specific," Jack said.

Banks nodded as her brows bunched together. Jack could only wonder what thoughts were swirling around in her head. She closed her notepad, replaced it in her purse, and sat up a little straighter.

"I think that's all I have for you, Doctors."

Madison said, "I'm sorry we couldn't be more helpful."

"You may have been more helpful than you know, Doctor. In my business, if you gather enough information from enough different sources, eventually the pieces begin to come together, and the truth reveals itself. It's probably not that much different from chasing down a tough diagnosis," she added with a modest smile.

Jack couldn't resist asking, "You didn't ask us any questions about the murders you're investigating."

"You're absolutely right, Dr. Wyatt. I didn't."

"I guess I'm still baffled by what two murders in Virginia that happened more than a year ago could have to do with a group of patients in Georgetown suffering from encephalitis?"

"Welcome to my world, Doctor because that's precisely what I'm trying to figure out." She went silent momentarily before adding, "I thought your meeting with Dr. Pike might have given you added insight into your patients' illness."

"That's an interesting comment," Madison said. "I'd ask you how you knew about the meeting, but I doubt you'd tell me."

"I wish I could, but I'm afraid you have your guidelines about disclosing information, and I have mine. But I will say this—and I may be repeating myself—I've spent a lot of time for the past year looking into two mysterious deaths, and the trail has taken me to the steps of the Georgetown Infirmary. Right now, I'm not prepared to write that off to a strange coincidence." Without waiting for a response, Banks stood up. "I appreciate you taking the time to speak with me, Doctors." She handed them each one of her business cards." If you should come across new information you feel comfortable sharing with me, please reach out."

"We can't promise you we'll be able to make that call," Madison said.

"You two strike me as quite bright. I'll remain optimistic you'll be able to find a way to do the right thing from a moral standpoint without violating any of your professional ethics."

She stepped away from the couch. Jack and Madison watched as she made her way across the lobby and exited the hotel.

"What the devil was that all about?" she asked.

Jack glanced down at the business card in his hand and flicked it a couple of times.

"I'm not sure, but I think you can add the FBI to those with concerns about the unusual circumstances surrounding this illness."

Chapter 43

SIXTH DAY

It was nine p.m., and Jack and Madison were seated at a table in the historic Off the Record Bar, each enjoying a perfectly prepared Manhattan. Madison continued to be engrossed by the dozens of framed political cartoons and caricatures covering the walls. They had shared a late dinner with Anise that went a little better than they both expected. After she left, they agreed she was a bit more resolved to the fact that her mother's illness would take more time to declare itself one way or the other. Seeming more optimistic than she'd been the last couple of days, Jack couldn't help but wonder if she were just getting better at disguising her true feelings.

"This is the first spare minute we've had, so let's get to it," Jack said, setting the file Dr. Pike had given him them on the table. Opening it, he separated the pages of each of the three case reports. Beginning with the symptoms, Pike's descriptions followed a time-line of each one of the patients' clinical courses. They included the limited lab work they'd had available to them some eighty-five years ago and a few x-ray reports. Pike's handwriting was excellent, and they had no trouble reading the notes. They continued to read as they discussed his findings.

"Well, there's no question they were all suffering from the same illness," Madison said. "Even though it was an accidental exposure, these men wound up as human lab rats. At least they all recovered."

"I'm sure the research team figured it would be foolish to look a gift horse in the mouth. They must have realized they could use the knowledge they gained from the technicians' illness to their advantage."

"We have no evidence that the work done by the government in the 1940s is in any way connected to what's going on with the Marsh employees. Since time is a major factor working against us, I'm not so sure how much of it we should spend trying to establish a connection."

"What makes you so sure?"

"Because I don't think it matters enough in our decision to treat for heavy metal toxicity. These case reports would make for a spirited medical discussion of an enigmatic illness, but I'm not sure it'll turn out to be much help to us," she said. "We don't even know if the toxins they studied at Horn ever made it out of the lab. And since the data they gathered isn't the type that winds up in the *New England Journal of Medicine*, I'm not sure we're any farther down the road than we were before we met with Dr. Pike.

"You may be right, but you have to admit that the one encouraging aspect is that all three of the men recovered. I know it's a stretch, but maybe it gives us some hope we'll see the same thing."

Jack briefly turned his attention back to rereading the description of the third man's symptoms when he realized that, in addition to sharing a group of neurologic symptoms, each of them had experienced one day of unremitting hiccups.

He continued, "With Elias in charge of the task group, things are very likely to get tougher for us. I agree with you that we're going to reach a point when we're going to have to decide whether we pitch Kristin on treating the Marsh patients for heavy metal poisoning or not." He held up a hand. "I'm just not sure we have enough corroborating laboratory evidence as yet to make that recommendation."

"Based on the patients continued decline, I think we have to go with what we have. Just how much longer can we keep kicking this can down the road? The measures for treating heavy metal toxicity go as far back as World War I, caring for soldiers affected by arsenic-based weapons. The various therapies have come a long way since then, and as Dr. Pike pointed out, they're well known to modern medical science."

"Are you suggesting we should advocate for empirical treatment of all the patients right now?" he asked her. "Maybe we should wait to see if Dr. Corsair comes up with anything confirmatory in her lab? It was at your behest that Dr. Pike agreed to ask one of his colleagues."

"I know, but the more I think about it, the more I'm convinced we don't have that kind of time. I'm can't get passed the fact that the antiviral therapy's a complete failure and that every one of our patients continues to get worse by the hour. To me, the conclusion we can draw from these two realities is obvious—it's time to act."

With an unexpressed thought settling into his head, Jack reached for his glass and took a slow sip of his iced tea. He knew the way Madison was looking at the medical aspects of the cases was spot on. Even so, his initial thought was to rein her in a little and gather additional information to strengthen their argument. He wasn't concerned about convincing Kristin of the advisability of moving forward with treatment — it was persuading Elias Rutledge and the other doctors to follow suit that had him beyond worried.

But the more he thought about it, the more he agreed with Madison that any further delay in instituting treatment for heavy metal poisoning could easily turn out to be a fatal error in judgment.

Chapter 44

Eighteen months after the Georgetown Infirmary had admitted its first patient, the Marsh Board of Trustees had presided over a ribbon-cutting ceremony to mark the opening of the hospital's ten-story state-of-the-art medical office building and simulator center used principally for the training of residents. As part of her recruitment package, Marsh had arranged for Kristin to be provided with a large corner office that she was given carte blanche to decorate. She had the talent to make it professional in appearance without crossing over into something overstated.

As she did more often than she cared to, she returned to her office to tackle the ever-enlarging stack of work that accumulated on her desk. On this particular evening, the time had gone by quickly, and before she knew it, it was close to eleven o'clock. She still had a couple of dozen emails to answer, but feeling beyond fatigued, she decided to call it a night.

After stretching her arms high over her head for a few seconds, she reached for her purse and came out from behind her desk. Grabbing her umbrella, she left her office with one small light on and stepped out into the corridor. The air in the hall was even chillier than it was in her office, prompting a light shiver to slip down her spine. Ever since she'd moved into her office, it had remained a complete mystery to her why Facilities kept the building so uncomfortably cold, especially at night.

She made her way down the faintly lit corridor. Due to the hour, the entire floor was blanketed by a stark silence. She didn't notice anybody else working late, but it wasn't the first time she'd been the last physician to leave. Even so, it still made her a little skittish to be there alone.

She continued down the hallway toward the elevators. When she was about halfway there, she heard the muted clang of the heavy metal door that accessed the stairwell. She took a hasty look over her shoulder, but in the scant light she couldn't see anybody. Still a little uneasy, she continued to move forward. But after a few seconds she stopped, and with her eyes squinted, she craned her neck and took a long look toward her office. This time she was certain she could make out the faint silhouette of a man standing at the far end of the hall, gazing through the large glass wall that formed the front of her office.

At first she thought it might be one of the security guards, but the minute he took a step back where the light was a little stronger, she instantly dismissed the possibility. He was wearing dark pants and what looked to be a hooded windbreaker. She instantly gulped a panicked breath. Before she could turn around, he looked right at her. Wasting no time, he started toward her at a deliberate pace. Convinced he was an intruder with no good intentions, a pulse of adrenaline streamed into her veins, whipping her heart with suffi-cient force to where she could feel each beat pulsating out of her chest and radiating into her neck.

With her only thought being to get to the elevator as quickly as possible, Kristin broke into a frenzied dash. A sudden flash of pain gripped her chest, clipping each breath she took. Terrified to slow down enough to steal another glimpse over her shoulder, she continued on. She felt as if she were trapped in a nightmare where time stood still, and no matter how hard she struggled to sprint, her legs were stuck in slow motion.

The moment she reached the elevator, she smacked the down

button and whirled around. Her eyes flashed down the hall. The man continued toward her, rapidly closing the distance between them. Striking the button over and over again, she kept her eyes fixed on him. For reasons she didn't understand, he slowed his pace and stared directly at her as if his intent was to taunt her.

A menacing smirk suddenly appeared on his face. If he intended to rob or harm her, Kristin wondered why he wasn't approaching more rapidly. It was almost as if he was finding enjoyment in prolonging her terror. Her phone was in a zippered pocket inside her bag. To get to it, she'd have to slide the bag off her shoulder. She knew she didn't have that much time. But what she did have sufficient time for was to grab the canister of pepper spray that she always kept in the large outside pocket.

He was now only about twenty feet away and still coming toward her at a steady but unhurried pace. She raised her eyes to the digital floor indicator above the cars. Just as she did, it switched to the seventh floor, and the doors rolled open. Jumping inside, she pressed her fingertip against the lobby button and prayed the doors would close before he reached her. With her entire body quaking, she readied the pepper spray.

Her heart was still hammering into her throat. It seemed like an eternity, but the doors finally started to roll closed. Their edges were a couple of inches away from slamming shut when she suddenly saw the man's hand, then his forearm, slide through the opening, preventing the doors from closing. The next thing she knew, they began to reverse direction. She knew she was within a few short seconds of him having her trapped in the elevator.

With her thumb on the actuator, Kristin raised the canister to eye level and lunged forward. She was in a perfect position when the doors opened sufficiently for her to see his face. In a split second, her thumb fully depressed the actuator. She prayed he'd jump backward, which would allow the doors to close and the car to descend to the lobby.

Her aim was true, as evidenced by the man's guttural groan that echoed in the elevator. But to her dismay, he held his position, reacting to the liquid irritant by rotating his head all the way to the right. Frantically, he pawed and rubbed at his eyes with one hand while keeping the doors open with the other. He appeared to be suffering the full effects of the pepper spray, but Kristin knew, even with his impaired vision, he'd be able to trap her against the back wall of the car. Her eyes darted back and forth. There was no way of getting past him. It was at that moment she took a small step to her right and stepped on the handle of her umbrella. While he was still rubbing at his eyes with the sleeve of his windbreaker, she leaned down and grabbed it from the floor.

Dropping his hand from his eyes, he started forward, widely swinging his open hand to detect anything in front of him. He took another step that placed him fully in the car with her, making it clear to Kristin she was seconds away from being cornered. She directed the metal tip of the umbrella squarely at his chest. Leaping forward, she drove the pointed tip into the center of his breastbone with every bit of strength she could muster. Before she could bring the umbrella back for a second thrust, the man was already screeching in pain and spinning toward the side of the cab. His momentum carried him into the wall, where he slid to his knees, gasping for air. In a blink of an eye, Kristin flew past him. Praying he wouldn't recover sufficiently to pursue her, she bolted for the stairwell.

As soon as she crashed through the stairwell door leading to the lobby, her eyes dashed around the area, desperately searching for a security guard. When she didn't spot one, she hurried out of the building and toward the hospital where there was always a police officer in the lobby working an off-duty detail. Kristin entered the lobby and immediately spotted the officer sitting at the security desk.

"There's an intruder in the medical office building," she said in a breathless voice. "He…he tried to attack me."

As the officer lifted her radio from her belt, she hurried out from behind the counter.

"Try and calm yourself, Doctor. Have a seat right here while I call this in." As soon as she requested assistance, she sat down in the chair next to Kristin. "Where was the last place you saw him?"

"The elevator on the seventh floor—he tried to trap me inside."

"Did he have a weapon?"

"I don't know…I didn't see one. I was able to use my pepper spray and get away."

"Do you remember what he was wearing?"

"Dark jeans and a hooded blue windbreaker. He was about six feet tall and had a full beard."

It was at that moment, when Kristin finally felt safe, that she broke down in tears. The officer placed her hand on her shoulder as she made a second call to the station to brief the dispatcher with the additional information.

Three minutes later, two cruisers with their blue and red lights flashing pulled up in front of the medical office building. By the time the officers reached the seventh floor, the man had recovered enough to drag himself to the back stairwell and flee the building.

A MILE AWAY, Regan Cullen sat in front of her television waiting for the man's call acknowledging that he'd successfully executed their plan. Her phone rang.

"It didn't exactly go to plan, but she got the message," he told her, recounting the events.

"So you never actually spoke to her?"

"No."

"If I'm understanding this correctly, I sent an ex–Special Ops guy on a relatively easy mission, and he winds up getting pepper-sprayed like a common mugger and harpooned by a Mary Poppins umbrella. Is that about it? Hell, I thought I was sending a pro. That sounds more like amateur hour."

"As I said, she got the message."

"How the hell do you know? Are you a mind reader? You just told me you didn't say a single word to her."

"She was sufficiently terrified. That was the plan. It wasn't a termination. I agree that it didn't go exactly as planned but I'm comfortable that I accomplished what I was supposed to."

"I could agree with you, but then we'd both be wrong," she told him. "As far as Dr. Hartzell knows, you could have been the bogey-man." With no interest in continuing the fruitless conversation, she said, "You bungled this badly, which makes us both look bad. That's it. Your bonehead blunder tonight ends it between us."

Throwing her phone against the couch, Regan walked over to the window wall and stared out over the wharf. Thinking about the shambles of the evening, she contemplated how she was going to break the news to Sol. When she'd first thought about dealing with Dr. Hartzell, it had crossed her mind to handle the problem person-ally. Having decided against the idea, she was now kicking herself for not following her instincts.

Chapter 45

SEVENTH DAY

Kristin typically did her best to arrive at the hospital an hour before her daily agenda began, to give herself time to stop at the hospital's coffee shop for a cappuccino, review her latest emails, and make any last-minute preparations for the many administrative and clinical meetings she would attend that day.

She had a little extra time this morning, and instead of grabbing the cappuccino and drinking it in her office, she decided to sit down and drink it in the coffee shop. She questioned the wisdom of that decision when, two minutes later, Aaron Steele strolled up to her.

"Busted," he said with a grin.

"Excuse me?"

"Somebody tipped me off you were a coffee addict and always stopped here before you started your day."

"You just can't trust anybody to keep your secrets these days." Since he'd gone out of his way to ambush her, Kristin suspected Aaron wasn't standing in front of her with something trivial on his mind. "May I buy you a coffee?"

"No thanks," he answered, pointing to the only other chair at the table. "But I wouldn't mind joining you for a few minutes... That is, if I won't be disturbing your private time."

"I haven't had any private time since high school. Have a seat, Aaron."

"Before we get into something else, how are you doing after that unfortunate experience last night? I'm surprised you didn't take the day off to recuperate a little."

"I thought about it but sitting around at home dwelling on it would have only made things worse. I decided I'd be better off working."

"I admire your strength. If that had happened to me I'm not sure I'd be doing as well as you obviously are."

"It was a pretty harrowing experience. I won't be working late in my office again, that's for sure."

"What have you heard from the police?"

"Not too much. The way he was dressed, the video surveillance wasn't much help."

"I've already had a chat with the hospital's upper echelon and given them a piece of my mind on the security company they contract with," he said with a wag of his finger. "If there's anything you need, please don't hesitate to let me know."

"Thanks, Aaron," she told him. "Now, you look like a man with something on his mind."

"I heard the intriguing news from Elias about the encephalitis patients possibly being sick because of some poison. Is that accurate?"

"It's a long shot, but in the interest of being complete, we're ruling it out."

His face tightened with doubt. "I need the inside word on this because I'm meeting with Erik and the rest of the leadership team later this morning to brief them. So I'd appreciate whatever additional information you have that I can share with them."

"There's not much more to it than what Elias told you. We're very focused on being thorough—an error in diagnosis will almost certainly lead to errors in treatment."

"I'm not a physician, so please bear with me: If the encephalitis were being caused by a toxin and not a virus, how did the folks at Fort Detrick discover this highly virulent virus in our patients' spinal fluid?"

"Maybe you should've been a doctor because that's a very logical question. The chance we're dealing with a lab error is fairly small. Again, we're just double-checking everything."

"For the purposes of my meeting this morning, am I correct in assuming your team's evaluation for some poisonous toxin…at least to this point…has been totally negative?"

"That's correct, but we don't have a test for every toxin out there," she answered. "Forgive me for asking, Aaron, but why is the C-suite getting so deep into the weeds on the medical details of this illness?"

He grinned. "Because they get deep into the weeds on just about everything. As far as my own precious butt is concerned, I have to be prepared to answer whatever they might ask."

"Why can't you simply tell them we're doing everything in our power to provide these individuals with the best possible care?"

"They already know that. But they also want to be assured that, whatever their fate might be, Marsh won't be held responsible. It's that simple." It wasn't that she was surprised by Aaron's answer, but she still found it disheartening on a purely visceral level. "I'm sure you understand that the company believes they're blameless in this matter. All of us on the executive committee are extremely anxious to put this unfortunate situation it in our rearview mirror as quickly as possible."

"I understand their concerns, but as physicians, we can't put these things on a timetable. We simply can't plan for everything, and we can't anticipate every possible change in an illness. If it's accountability that the powers that be are uber-focused on…well, I can't and won't make any guarantees until we have all the answers."

He pushed his palms together. His face hardened, betraying his mounting exasperation.

"Kristin, try to remember, you're not only a doctor—you're also a high-ranking member of this organization, and we're expecting you to conduct yourself with that in mind. I guess what I'm trying to say is that I need you to be a team player."

"Since I'm not sure what that might entail, I'll do my best but I can't make that promise. I'm not trying to appear uncooperative or stubborn, but I thought Marsh hired me as physician above everything else."

"So what are you trying to say?" he asked with a plastic smile.

"Isn't it obvious? I'm not going to do anything that's morally or ethically corrupt in the name of facilitating the company's business or political agenda. We're all responsible for culpability and accountability. My position doesn't mean I'm not a team player."

"Sometimes, I feel as if you have a funny way of showing it."

"Which you've already demonstrated by removing me from leading the task group," she responded, raising her hand. "Of late, it seems like the conflict between what's good for Marsh and the oath I took the day I graduated from medical school are constantly at loggerheads. We're still facing an enormous problem, Aaron. The last thing I need from our leadership is added pressure."

"On the other hand, maybe a return to reality will help you unmuddy the waters."

"I beg your pardon?" she said, feeling her nostrils flaring. To this point Aaron had only moved the line, but he was now getting dangerously close to stepping over it.

"Worldwide, this organization has over a hundred and seventy thousand employees. That makes us larger than most cities. Every day a certain number of those people face a major crisis, and oftentimes that crisis leads to death," he explained in a tone that had stiffened with displeasure. "We're a compassionate and caring company, but we also have a mission that presents us with certain operational imperatives. You speak to me about our responsibilities? What about our responsibility to help maintain the security of this country by expertly fulfilling our defense contracts? Whatever's going to happen to those patients on the fourth floor is going to happen. Certainly, you're not too obtuse to understand that."

"Take caution in the way you speak to me, Aaron. I don't appreciate your abusive behavior, and I assure you, I won't hesitate to act if I believe you're creating a hostile work environment."

"I apologize. That's obviously not my intention," he informed her calmly. "Perhaps you can think of it this way. I'm asking you for a favor. Someday you may be in a similar situation and need my help for something that's important to you."

She gently bit her lip before responding. "I'm not a big believer in quid pro quo, and I won't sell my soul to the devil. What I'm saying is that I'd sooner resign my position than be indebted or beholden to anybody in the way you're implying."

Kristin crumpled her napkin and dropped it on his side of the table.

"And regarding your executive staff meeting today, please feel free to express my feelings to the entire room. If anybody wishes to have a follow-up conversation with me, I'll make myself immediately available…and, Aaron, anytime you get the notion that this might not be the best job for me, well…just like you oftentimes say, the door to my office is always open."

And then, without so much as a look in his direction, she marched out of the coffee shop.

Chapter 46

Once Nicole had made her decision to accept the position at Marsh and move back to the United States, one of the first items on her to-do list was to select a school for Anise to attend. When a friend told her about Rochambeau French International School in Bethesda, the choice became an easy one. It was a nationally renowned preparatory school offering a French international curriculum. Being quite familiar with the French system of education, Anise had no trouble adapting to Rochambeau's approach to education. It was a perfect fit.

It was a dreary afternoon, and having no after-school activities, Anise left school and headed directly for the student parking lot. Two days after her seventeenth birthday, she'd taken her driving test and passed it with flying colors. Nicole, confident in her daughter's highly responsible attitude toward driving, had presented her with the keys to a new dark-gray SUV.

Anise made her way to the far end of the parking lot, her preferred location for avoiding scratches and dents to her car by her less careful classmates. She was just about to open the door and climb in when Regan approached.

"Hi, Anise," she said with a welcoming smile. She immediately suffered a brain cramp as she struggled to place the pleasant woman. Her first thought was that she might be a new teacher who for some reason knew her name, although seeing teachers in the student lot was an uncommon occurrence. "Nice SUV. You're a lucky girl. I didn't get my first car until after I finished college," Regan said, running her hand along the side of the vehicle. "How do you like it so far?"

Stalling for time, hoping she'd suddenly remember the woman's name, she said, "It's perfect. We couldn't have made a better choice."

"I was so sorry to learn that your mom's so terribly ill. I wish her only the best."

"Thank you. Do you know her?"

"We were introduced once, but I doubt she'd remember. But I'm very familiar with your father and the wonderful work he does. I also know of Dr. Shaw, your soon-to-be stepmom."

Anise was surprised at the woman's comment but said nothing. As far as she knew, their plans to get married were still confidential. Anise finally gave up the ghost and admitted, "I'm so embarrassed to admit this, but I can't recall your name. Have we met?"

"No, we haven't, and my name's really not important. But as long as we're talking, you should know that, while I'm very worried about your mother, I'm more worried about you and your father. That's why I came here today. I wanted to speak to you about it."

"Excuse me?" Anise said, overtaken by uncertainty. "Are you a doctor?"

"Heavens no. I faint at the sight of my own blood," she said with a hint of a grin. But just as quickly as it appeared, it fell from her face, being replaced by a more solemn look. "Actually, my job entails many things, like making sure people don't meddle into matters that don't concern them."

"I'm sorry, but I don't have the first clue what you're talking about." It wasn't in Anise's DNA to be easily intimidated or to back away from a thorny situation. She had no intention of bowing out of the conversation by inventing some lame excuse to leave.

"It's really not that complicated," Regan said. "Sometimes very intelligent people who get wrapped up in what they're doing don't see the big picture. Don't get me wrong. Your dad's a great doctor, and he's doing everything in his power to help your mom. But there's something I'm going to need your help with."

"My help?" she asked in a voice that dripped with annoyance.

"Calm down, Anise. I'm simply saying you'll be an enormous help to your mom's recovery if you simply tell your dad to focus on curing her and the other Marsh patients of their encephalitis and nothing else."

"I was under the impression that's what he was doing."

"I hope so, but we all could use a reminder from time to time. So if you simply share with your father what I just told you, I promise you he'll understand. Can you do that, please?"

"And, if I say no?"

"I wouldn't recommend that. Think of my request as something that's for your benefit."

"That makes no sense. I thought you were worried about my mom. Why don't you tell him yourself, if this is so important?"

Regan smiled. "Ask your dad that question. He'll understand why this little piece of advice has to come from you."

Anise stood there dumbfounded, suspecting that the woman had barely grazed the truth with anything she'd said.

"Drive carefully," she said as she strolled away. "The number of car accidents involving teenagers in the DC area is frightening."

Chapter 47

Because of her imperiled pregnancy, Madison had been keeping a special eye on Lori Somersby. She and Jack generally took some time in the late afternoon, Jack to check on Nicole and Madison to check on Lori. One of the few things that Madison remained optimistic about was the condition of the baby. While Lori continued to battle her disease, the baby managed to hold her own.

As usual, Madison had seen Lori on morning rounds. There was an abundance of clinical evidence that her condition was critical and, not surprisingly, that the antiviral medication was failing to help. She remained on the ventilator, and the medications necessary to maintain her blood pressure and support her vital organs were being increased with each passing hour.

Madison had just started her exam of Lori when Gretchen came through the door. She set her briefcase on the table and walked to the bedside.

"How's she doing, Dr. Shaw?"

"She's not quite as strong as she was yesterday or earlier today, but her vital signs have remained stable." The two eventualities that Madison feared the most were respiratory failure and sepsis. That combination would almost certainly spell the end of things.

"And the baby?" Gretchen asked.

"She's experiencing the expected amount of stress. It's obviously not what we want to see, but on the other hand, it could be a lot worse. Right now, I'd say she's stable. As we've talked about, if Lori's condition worsens, it could definitely impact the baby's course as well."

"Have you made any progress in finding a treatment for the virus?"

"The two antiviral drugs we've tried don't seem to be working. All the physicians are going to meet later today to consider either adding another medication or completely changing the antiviral drug regimen we've been using."

After a few moments, tears pooled in Gretchen's eyes and she said in just above a whisper, "This woman's the love of my life, Dr. Shaw. This may sound strange, but I still can't believe any of this is really happening."

"The only thing you can do right now is stay the course and not give up hope."

An adoring look appeared on Gretchen's face. "Don't worry. I won't let that happen. Every day I walk in here expecting to see Lori sitting up in bed, wide-eyed, fingers flashing away on her phone playing Candy Crush. She just can't seem to get enough of the silly game."

"I have tons of friends and colleagues who've fallen victim to the same addiction. I'm not sure I totally understand it."

Madison spent the next few minutes with Gretchen giving her a more detailed account of Lori's condition. The look in Gretchen's eyes betrayed her struggle with the gravity of the situation.

"I know you're doing your best to sound optimistic, Dr. Shaw, but every aspect of Lori's illness is getting worse. All the families have gotten pretty close. We talk all the time, and none of us has much hope left. I'd say we've shifted to preparing for the inevitable. From my layperson perspective, the only thing in this entire illness that's gotten better is her hiccups."

Instantly making the connection to Dr. Pike's patients, Madison blinked with surprise. "I've been over Lori's chart numerous times. I don't remember any mention of her

having the hiccups."

"I've spoken to so many doctors since Lori was admitted. Most of that time I've been in a semi state of shock, so to tell you the truth, I can't remember the specifics of what I told anybody."

"Do you recall when she had the hiccups and for how long they lasted?"

"The first I remember noticing them was the morning of the second day. They were pretty intense for about a day and then just kind of stopped." Gretchen paused. "I'm getting the feeling you think I should have mentioned this sooner?"

"Not really. It's probably just a coincidental finding."

"I'm glad to hear that," she told Madison.

"Do you have any other questions for me?"

"Only, when do you think you'll be stopping in again?"

"Tomorrow morning."

"I'll be here...and, Dr. Shaw, I know I can be abrupt, and I sometimes forget my manners. If you've noticed it, I hope you understand it's the situation and not my nature. Lori's illness has me so on edge I can't sleep, eat, or do my job." Madison watched as Gretchen's gaze became disconnected. "If I lose Lori and our baby, I...I don't know what I'll do."

"I have to believe we're going to figure this thing out and come up with a way to treat it. I can't allow myself to lose that hope."

Gretchen gave her a hug. "Thanks for everything, Dr. Shaw. I think I'm starting to believe you. I'll see you tomorrow morning."

The moment Madison left the room, she called Jack.

"I just checked on Lori. She and the baby are about the same, but I'm very anxious to talk to you about something. Can you meet me?"

"Sure. I'm in the middle of checking Nicole. I need about twenty minutes. Is that okay?"

"That's fine. It's a beautiful afternoon for a walk. Why don't we head down to the park and talk along the way?"

"Sure."

"I'll meet you in the lobby in twenty-five minutes," she said.

You sound pretty anxious. Is everything okay?"

"Everything's fine. I'll see you in twenty-five minutes…and Jack," she added sternly. "I mean a normal person's twenty-five minutes."

"Ouch," he told her.

⊏━⊐

WHILE JACK WAS TURNING his attention to doing an eye examination, he couldn't help but wonder what was on Madison's mind. He finished his exam and replaced the ophthalmoscope in its case. He reached for Nicole's hand to check her fingernails. The presence of the Mees lines had been a key finding on her physical examination. They were still present, and they hadn't changed in their extent or appearance.

While he was gently replacing her hand on the bed, Jack thought he felt something on the pad of one of her fingertips. Rolling her hand over, he took a careful look at the area of interest. The lesion was barely visible, perhaps only two millimeters in size, and slightly raised. It was most consistent with a partially healed minor wound. He didn't think much of the finding until it crossed his mind to have a look at her other fingertips. To his surprise, there was a similar lesion on each of Nicole's fingertip pads. Taking a step back, he sank into deep thought.

To his knowledge, there was no association between viral encephalitis and minute healing lesions of the fingertips. He was doubtful any of the doctors would have noticed them by just looking at the patients' hands, and he considered himself fortunate to have discovered one by pure serendipity. The obvious question popped into his head—did any of the other patients have the same finding as Nicole on the pads of their fingers?

Jack checked the time. He still had fifteen minutes before he was to meet Madison. Before heading downstairs to the lobby, he briefly stopped in each Marsh patient's room and examined his or her fingertip pads. To his surprise, each patient except Jordan Hinzman demonstrated the lesions on all their fingers. In his case, the only place Jack could confirm them was on his index fingers. He had no idea why.

He walked off the unit and headed toward the stairwell, his mind churning like a cyclone. It was an unmistakable fact that there was no association of fingertip lesions and viral encephalitis, which left him wondering what could have caused the lesions. The most obvious possibility was that they were caused by direct contact with something.

He felt a flutter in his gut as his mind continued to shuffle through the possible causes of the lesions. His inner voice was telling him in no uncertain terms that among the possibilities was the smoking gun they were so desperately searching for.

Chapter 48

Jack and Madison exited the Infirmary and made their way south along Wisconsin Avenue with the plan of continuing on until they reached the Georgetown Waterfront Park.

Jack said, "Before you tell me what's on your mind, I wanted to let you know that I had a rather worrisome conversation with Anise. It seems she was approached in her student parking lot by a woman she didn't recognize. The woman instructed her to tell me to confine my role regarding the Marsh patients to matters that are purely medical in nature. It seems she had quite a bit of information about Nicole and me. She also knew that you and I are planning on getting married."

"Did she come out and directly threaten Anise?"

"Not in so many words, but it may have been there by innuendo. I guess it's possible she was just bluffing."

"Who would do something like that?"

"I don't know, but I guess there are a few possibilities. Anise's experience is just another disturbing reminder that we don't know anything about the non-clinical circumstances surrounding these cases."

"How did she take the whole thing. Is she afraid?"

With a slow shake of his head, Jack said, "A little maybe, but she doesn't cower from anything very easily. I think it's more that she's riled somebody would try to strong-arm her."

"But why would somebody do that?"

"I don't know. I'd say, whoever this woman was, she was shooting for intimidation more than anything. The question is why?"

"Maybe it has something to do with the story beginning to get its fair share of media attention, or what about some disgruntled family member who has a strange way of expressing her dissatisfaction?" With a shrug, she added, "The world's full of lunatics whose behavior can't be accounted for. The question is, what are you going to do about it?"

"Obviously, for myself, I'm not going to back away from anything related to the care of Nicole and the other Marsh patients. I assume you feel the same way. As for Anise, I have a couple of ideas."

"Whatever you do, you can't terrify her in the process. Are you thinking about sending her out of town?"

"Anise is seventeen and extremely headstrong. There's no way she's going to leave Nicole."

"Would it really be her decision?"

"She'd make it her decision. She's not going to stay someplace outside the city voluntarily, and I can't send her somewhere that will keep her under lock and key."

"That only leaves two options," she said. "Either you do nothing, or you do something here in DC."

"I agree."

"Instead of wasting a lot of time thinking about it," Madison began slowly, "why don't you just call Mike? Because, in the end, that's what you're going to do anyway."

"Believe me, that was the first thing that occurred to me."

"That's what lifelong best friends are for. You two would jump in front of a speeding train for each other. More important than anything, Mike and Tess love Anise as much as they do their own kids."

Seeing no need for further conversation or contemplation, he reached for his phone and called Mike.

"Hey, buddy. How's life in sunny South Florida?" Jack asked.

"If I were ever there, I'm sure it would be wonderful, but right now I'm in Panama."

"Stop buying up companies all over the world and try putting your feet up at home for a few days."

"Tess would murder me if I was around that much."

Jack chuckled. "And what would you do without that next multi-billion-dollar deal that's right around the corner?"

"Tess told me the other day the only thing that sets my hair on fire is playing real Monopoly. So what's going on up in Washington? Is Nicole getting better?"

"She's still pretty sick, but we're working on some things we hope will work."

"I assume Madison's with you."

"Every step of the way."

"And Anise…how's she holding up?"

"Still hanging on by her fingernails."

The call descended into silence for a few seconds. Mike finally said, "I doubt you called me for medical advice, and since you're my closest friend in the world, why don't you tell me what's on your mind?"

"I'm worried about Anise, and I may need your help."

Jack then spent a few minutes bringing Mike up to speed on her strange encounter at school and his concern about her safety.

"Okay, there's an easy solution here," Mike said without a second thought. "I'll have Tess pack a bag, and I'll put her on the jet later today and send her up to DC to stay with Anise until things straighten out. I'm on my way to Buenos Aires from here for a few days, but I'll be home by the weekend. As soon as I take care of a couple of things in Miami, I'll head up there and join you guys."

"I'm not sure that's completely nec—"

"Necessary? Kind of like it wasn't necessary for you to cut your vacation short in the Caribbean, come to South Florida, and save Tess's life? Let's not go there, okay?"

"Thanks, Mike. I don't know what to say."

"It'll work out great. Tess and Anise love each other. And you and I will have a chance to catch up. It hasn't escaped my attention or Tess's that you turned us down cold the last two times we asked you and Madison to go away with us."

"It's not necessary to remind me. It's Madison's job to berate me about my workaholic tendencies. We'll do something in the spring. I promise."

"Great. We'd love that. As soon as we get off the phone, I'll call Tess and start making the arrangements. She should be there some-time this evening. As soon as they land, she'll go directly to Nicole's building."

"They?"

"She'll be traveling with Griffin. He's our personal concierge and principal."

"Principal? Isn't that code for a bodyguard?"

"I prefer to think of him as a personal assistant with highly developed martial arts skills. He's a cross between Rambo and the guy from Taken. Believe me, if anybody comes anywhere near Tess or Anise, it'll be the sorriest day of their life. I'm out of town a lot and I sleep easier with Griffin keeping an eye on the family. I can't wait to see you, buddy."

"Same here."

Jack replaced the phone in its holder.

"Sounds like that problem's taken care of," Madison said.

"That's why we always used to call him Mike the Machine," he said, looking down the river at the Francis Scott Key Bridge. "Now that I've used up almost our entire walk on my problem, tell me what's on your mind."

Madison began the conversation by filling Jack in on her discovery that Lori had experienced hiccups for a full day before they spontaneously subsided. He, too, didn't need to be reminded that, according to Dr. Pike's notes, the three individuals stationed at Horn Island who were accidently exposed to one of the toxins all had hiccups for a day.

"So what do you think?" she asked him.

"Did any of our other patients experience hiccups early on in their illness?"

"I haven't had a chance to check yet, but I don't recall seeing it mentioned in any of the medical records. As soon as we get back to the hospital, I'm going to recheck the patients' charts just to make sure. And when we make afternoon rounds, I'm going to ask all the family members directly if they recall any episodes of hiccups."

Jack said, "If you do confirm it, it would be another strong indication that the Marsh patients aren't suffering from viral encephalitis. When we add it to the other clinical findings that argue against a diagnosis it obviously strengthens our case that we've been barking up the wrong tree."

They stopped at the corner, waited for the crosswalk light to turn green, and then crossed the street. Once they entered the park, they made their way down to the Potomac River.

Jack said, "As long as we're on the topic of diagnostic errors and making a case against encephalitis, there's something else I should fill you in on."

"Shoot."

"After you called, I discovered something interesting on Nicole's exam. Since I had a few minutes before I had to meet you, I checked the other patients for the same finding."

"Don't keep me in suspense."

"Except for one, they all have minute lesions on their fingertips. They're slightly raised, which makes them palpable. If I didn't know better, I'd say they're tiny healing abrasions."

"You said there was one exception."

"Jordan Hinzman only has the lesions on his index fingers."

Madison slowed her pace, looked at him through cautious eyes, and then stopped dead in her tracks. "Are you absolutely sure about that?"

"Of course."

She could barely contain the broad smile that landed on her face. "So Mr. Hinzman's a hunt-and-peck guy."

"Excuse me?"

"You're the one who asked for more proof that the Marsh

patients aren't suffering from encephalitis— well, this is it…you found it." Jack went silent, standing there with a blank look on his face. She took his hand, gave it a squeeze, and hurried him along. "I don't think you're connecting the dots here, buddy. That's not like you."

Chapter 49

EIGHTH DAY

Because of their ongoing exhaustion, Jack and Madison stole an extra hour of sleep before finally getting out of bed. They were still in their room talking and getting ready when his phone rang.

He crossed his fingers and held them up for Madison to see. When he checked the caller ID, he uncrossed them and gave her a thumbs-up.

"It's Dr. Pike," he said, as he accepted the call and activated the speaker function.

"Good morning, Dr. Pike."

"Good morning, Jack. Are you and Madison available to meet with me this morning? I tried reaching Kristin as well, but I had no luck."

"Of course. When will you be available?"

"There's no time like the present."

Understanding the potential importance of a meeting with Dr. Pike, Jack said, "That's fine. Considering the morning traffic, it'll probably take Madison and I about an hour to get to your home."

"That won't be necessary. I'm already in D. C."

"In that case, where would you like to meet?"

"How does the lobby of your hotel sound?"

"That's kind of you to offer, but Madison and I are happy to meet you wherever you say to make it more convenient for you."

"In that case, let's definitely make it in your lobby, because that's where I am. You'll find me sitting on a black leather couch next to an enormous potted plant."

"We're almost ready to leave the room. How about if we meet you in ten minutes?"

"Actually, I'm feeling kind of hungry so, on second thought, let's meet in the restaurant."

"That sounds perfect. We'll see you there." Jack ended the call and turned to Madison.

"This sounds very promising. I doubt he'd come all this way if he had nothing of significance to share with us."

"He's a pretty eccentric guy. You may be being overly optimistic in assuming he can be relied upon to do things the way most people do."

"I guess we're about to find that out."

Ten minutes later, Jack and Madison walked into the restaurant and were escorted to Dr. Pike's table. He'd already gone through the buffet line and was busily working on a breakfast that would have satisfied a defensive lineman on game day.

"Good morning," Madison said, holding back a smile when she noted he was wearing the same faded cargo jeans he'd worn at their first meeting. She couldn't help but wonder if they were his only pair or if they were one of many that hung in his closet.

He raised his fork and gestured with it. "I'm happy to wait if you folks want to go through the line and grab something to eat."

"We decided to skip breakfast this morning," Jack said.

Between rapid bites of his blueberry pancakes, he said, "Dr. Corsair called me at five this morning. She'd been up all night with a couple of her lab techs working on the specimens you sent her. I know her pretty well, and she's generally a fairly calm individual, but she was pretty excited this morning. Without boring you with too many of the details, they ran a lot of tests but paid particular attention to those that use mass spectrometry," he informed them, stopping his breakfasting long enough to scrub his hands on his napkin. "She was convinced that none of the commonly recognized heavy metals were present in any of the samples. However, she was reasonably certain there was evidence of some heavy metal contamination in the blood and perhaps the hair samples."

"Does she think she identified was something new?" Madison asked.

"So it would seem."

"How specific was she regarding what she found?"

"She didn't have a lot of details. All she'd commit to was that they found chemical evidence of a substance that had properties in the heavy metal family. She said her best guess was that it had been derived from a mixture of known heavy metals—likely including thallium."

"Which would imply it's not a metal found naturally in the environment," Jack said.

Pike raised his coffee cup in a mock toast and winked. "You said it, not me. She told me she'd never seen anything quite like it, if that helps." Holding his next thought briefly, he looked at each of them in turn. "If you don't mind me asking, just how familiar are you two with treating heavy metal poisonings?" When they didn't respond quickly enough for his liking, he continued. "Before you two mastermind a plan that leads you across a crocodile-infested river, let me share a few facts with you."

"Please do," Madison was quick to say.

"As I mentioned the first time we spoke, the mainstay of treatment remains chelating agents. We have a lot of them available to us now, but they all work basically the same way, which is binding to a particular heavy metal, forming a compound with it, and then eliminating it by the body excreting it in the urine. As physicians, we sometimes forget that chelation therapy is hardly without possible complications. The most serious ones are damage to both the kidneys and the liver. Other things have been added to the treatment protocols, such as antioxidants and some other more creative techniques. If you're dealing with thallium poisoning, Prussian blue is the principal therapeutic weapon."

Madison realized his explanation was on the elementary side, but she wasn't going to lose the opportunity of taking Dr. Pike one level higher.

"I realize you don't have a lot to go on, but what's your take on Dr. Corsair's findings?"

"I'll give this to you with the gloves off. I believe you're dealing with heavy metal poisoning at the Infirmary. I suspect it's not naturally occurring and that there's an excellent chance you're not going to cure anybody with standard chelation therapy alone." The conversation came to an abrupt end. Both Jack and Madison realized there was wisdom in Pike's prediction. He then said flatly, "I'm afraid you'll have to find another way to deal with this problem." Raising his eyes from his plate, he added in earnest, "Other than that, I'm afraid there's nothing else I can tell you."

"Thanks for all your assistance, Dr. Pike," Jack told him.

"I hope Dr. Corsair and I have been able to help you. I'm going to sit for a while and finish my breakfast, but don't let me hold you up," he said with a wink and a wave of his hand. "Something tells me you two are going to be busier than a couple of one-armed wallpaper hangers today at Georgetown Infirmary."

Jack and Madison slowly got up from the table and exited the dining room. As soon as they reached the lobby, Jack reached for his phone and called Kristin to arrange an urgent meeting.

"That sounds fine," Jack said to her. "And thank you. We'll see you then."

"What's the plan?" Madison asked.

"Her schedule's packed all the way into tonight. She's got a small window of time where she can see us this afternoon, but she was counting on working out for about thirty minutes. She said if we don't mind, we can talk while she's on the treadmill, so we're meeting her at three at the Infirmary's exercise center."

Madison grinned as they continued across the lobby and exited the hotel. "Dr. Pike's really something," she said. "When I compile my official list of the most original and interesting people I've ever met, he may very well turn out to be numero uno."

Chapter 50

Jack and Madison walked into the hospital's state-of-the-art workout center and spotted Kristin immediately. She had already started her time on the microgravity treadmill. Jack recalled going through a short-lived phase last year when he'd worked out on a daily basis. After watching the energy Kristin was exerting, he could easily see why'd he given up exercise for Dunsany's Chess.

"How's the workout going?" Madison asked.

"Not too bad."

"How are you feeling?"

"I assume you're referring to my unexpected altercation of the other night."

"It did cross my mind, but if you'd rather not talk about it…"

"I'm happy to talk about it," she began without a particle of hesitation. "Growing up, I had four brothers. I was the only girl, and they were all older than I was. They loved me and hovered over me like four helicopters, but when we were home, they constantly tormented me. It made a survivor out of me. I was plenty scared, but maybe less than most other people would've been."

Madison made no attempt to conceal the amused grin that appeared on her face.

"I don't have the first clue what that asshole had in mind the other night. Maybe, for reasons that exceed my understanding, he got the feeling he was just trying to scare me. Whatever his sick, twisted reason was, it makes no difference. He's not going to send me cowering into some corner." She shook her head and added, "If I let that goon intimidate me, then he wins. My plan is to continue to do my job to the best of my ability. If he's dumb enough to try anything else, I'll beat his sorry ass into next week again."

Madison cleared her throat while at the same time Jack bit his lip.

"I was telling Jack a couple of days ago that you didn't strike me as somebody who sugarcoats things."

Kristin laughed and left the topic behind.

"I'm still trying to get used to this new treadmill. I'm not sure, but I think I'm gaining on it." She slowed her pace. "Before you get started with what's on your minds, I assume you're aware that we lost Carson Buckman late this morning. They coded him for forty minutes but couldn't get him back."

"We were in the hospital when it happened," Jack said.

"It looks like we're getting pushed to the wall to make certain decisions, so tell me about your meeting with Dr. Pike, because I have a feeling that's what you're here about."

Madison began by sharing Dr. Corsair's findings with Kristin. She then went on to explain that she and Jack were now convinced that some form of heavy metal poisoning was responsible for the illness and that the only rational thing to do was start treatment immediately.

With cautious restraint in her eyes, Kristin said, "At the risk of sounding obtuse, I just want to make sure you two are saying that you feel the clinical data is strong enough to recommend we treat all the patients blindly for heavy metal poisoning…even though we don't have a single assay that's identified one."

"I'm not sure we're comfortable with the blindly part, but we're confident it's the most logical next step," she said.

"Jack?" Kristin said.

"I'd take it one step further and say it's the only next step."

"Since we first spoke, I've done a little reading on the topic. I was surprised to learn that there have been all kinds of complications associated with chelation therapy—some serious, some even fatal."

"We understand that, but we don't feel as if we have a choice," Jack responded without a single qualm. "Dr. Corsair's finding may not be definitively make the case, but it's pretty damn close."

"And Dr. Pike agrees with the recommendation to begin therapy?"

"He agrees," Jack said.

"I see. Is he willing to make that official?"

Madison answered, "As you recall, we never asked him to make any of his impressions or recommendations official."

"I know that, but I was thinking it might help us convince the other members of the task group to buy into the idea. I'm a naturally optimistic person, but we may be reaching for something that's well beyond our grasp. I haven't taken a straw poll, but I'd say most of the physicians feel viral encephalitis is the correct diagnosis, and we're already doing everything in our power to treat these people. They may see embarking on a new and questionable treatment as a desperation move that could do more harm than good."

"Letting these patients die and using the *we did everything we could* rationalization would be a travesty," Madison insisted. "For god's sake, they have to realize it's too early for them to wave the white flag." From the growing intensity in her voice, Jack could easily sense Madison's growing exasperation. She went on, "I think we're obligated to at least make our feelings known to the other doctors. If they don't agree that treating for heavy metal toxicity is the only hope our patients have…well, there may be nothing more we can do. So I suggest we remain optimistic and give this final swing at the piñata our best shot."

Kristin said, "The one thing in our favor is that neither Elias Rutledge nor the task group is empowered to make this decision. Their role is purely an advisory one. The medical staff bylaws are clear on this topic, which means we have to get Connie Postalwaite involved. She serves as both our chief medical officer and director of the Division of Pulmonary Medicine."

"What can we expect from her?" Madison asked.

"If Connie perceives an obvious preference among the members of the task group, it's likely she'll go along with their wishes. If she's unpersuaded, then the ultimate decision to offer the treatment to the affected patients and their families is hers to make." After pausing for a couple of seconds, she added, "I can tell you that her decision will weigh heavily on how strong a case we make."

"I'm not sure we can ask much more than that," Jack said. "So what's next?"

"I'll give Connie a call and let her know what's going on. She has the option of calling a meeting of all the interested parties, or she can opt to speak individually with whomever she chooses."

"Which way do you think she'll go?" Madison asked.

"I know her pretty well. It's ninety percent she'll call a meeting. I'll let you guys know as soon as I have any information." Kristin got off the treadmill, grabbed a towel, and dabbed her face. In a muted voice, she confessed, "If there were a bar around here, I'd sit down and order a stiff drink."

Chapter 51

NINTH DAY

Jack and Madison were aware there were mixed feeling among the members of the physicians regarding the wisdom of abandoning their current diagnosis of adenovirus encephalitis and changing course to what some would consider a Hail Mary solution to the problem. The naysayers were likely to express their belief that the idea was reckless because there was no way to rule out the possibility of a spontaneous recovery. They'd insist that a critically ill patient destined to recover on their own might be robbed of that possibility if subjected to an unnecessary and aggressive therapy that had no hope of improving their condition.

As Kristin had predicted, Connie Postalwaite decided to set up a meeting to hear both sides of the argument. She'd invited all ten members of the physician task group, two of Georgetown Infirmary's ranking hospital administrators, and Aaron Steele, to sit in as Marsh's eyes and ears. She had considered a larger group but ultimately decided it would be a more productive meeting if the group was kept to a manageable number of attendees. Connie was a fair-minded, quick-on-the-uptake woman who understood how to pick her battles. In her role as chief medical officer, her fellow physicians were comfortable approaching her about all manner of problems and viewed her as the type of colleague who led by example.

There wasn't a lot of socializing or lollygagging immediately prior to the meeting. Everybody in attendance had been advised on the single agenda item in advance and understood the gravity of the situation. Upon entering the conference room, most said a polite hello and quickly found their seat around the conference table.

At precisely eight a.m., Connie called the meeting to order.

"I want to thank everyone for arranging their schedule to attend this morning's meeting. Let me begin by saying that I understand we have a difference of opinion regarding the treatment of these patients. But if there's one thing we can all agree upon, it's that time is of the essence. Therefore, I can assure everybody that by this evening one thing will be true that may not be true right now. We will be united in our treatment plan. Now's the time for a professional discussion, but when this meeting ends, so does that opportunity. It's not fair to our patients to have any dissension or second-guessing. Everybody gets on board with the treatment plan and does everything in her or his power to execute it."

She stopped and looked up and down the long conference table. "Are there any questions?"

When no one asked to be recognized, Connie continued, "Good. Let's move on then. I've been thoroughly briefed regarding the possibility of an alternative diagnosis. Elias Rutledge, as the one in charge of the group, has informed me that he and several other members who are strongly in favor of staying the course and avoiding any change in treatment. Dr. Hartzell disagrees. I'd therefore like to begin by giving her the opportunity to explain to us why she's convinced we've made an error in diagnosis and should alter our therapy."

Elias came to his feet. "I'd like to say something first that I believe will save us all a lot of time."

Connie looked at Kristin who nodded in approval.

"That's fine, Elias. Go ahead."

"If Dr. Hartzell would simply provide us with laboratory confirmation that our patients are suffering from heavy metal poisoning, I'm sure all of us would be totally supportive of beginning chelation therapy. However, if she cannot do so, I'd like to point out that treating a patient for heavy metal toxicity without confirmation of the disease being present is not only unheard of in modern medicine but would almost certainly be grounds for a medical malpractice action."

Kristin nodded. "Dr. Rutledge is correct. The routine toxicology reports we have don't identify a specific heavy metal."

Rutledge was quick to press his point. "We have a toxicologist on staff right here at the Infirmary who we consulted. Perhaps Dr. Hartzell could remind us of what his conclusions were."

"Dr. Rivers' evaluation failed to identify a specific toxic substance."

"Just to be clear, Kristin, I assume you're referring to a heavy metal."

"I'm referring to any toxin," she said.

Elias grinned as if he'd just won the Maryland lottery, raising his spindly hands to chest level with his palms up as if he were speaking the obvious. "I'm just wondering what specific poison Dr. Hartzell suspects is making these patients deathly ill yet has been able to elude Dr. Rivers, our laboratory, and an outside lab of Dr. Hartzell's choosing?"

"There's no additional information available. Since Dr. Wyatt and Dr. Shaw are in a better position than I am to answer that question, I'll ask them to respond to Dr. Rutledge."

Unable to temper his predilection for interrupting, Elias said, "I think that we're all aware the three of you have been consulting with Dr. Ralph Pike. He's not on our medical staff, nor has he been officially consulted by a physician who is. His opinion should therefore have no influence on the decisions we make here today."

Connie spoke up. "For goodness' sake, Elias. This isn't a court of law. And I, for one, am very much interested in the opinion of a physician of Dr. Pike's knowledge, experience, and national reputation. I am equally interested in what you have to say, but I'd appreciate it if you'd hold your questions and comments until we've heard from Drs. Wyatt and Shaw." She turned, set her eyes on Jack and Madison, and then nodded in their direction.

From his seat, Jack said, "As Dr. Rutledge mentioned, we consulted with Dr. Pike regarding our concerns about the possibility our patients are suffering from heavy metal poisoning," His voice was as assured as his manner was direct. "He agreed there was substantial reason for concern. He offered to ask Dr. Jenna Corsair for her assistance. Dr. Corsair's facility is one of the most comprehensive toxicology labs in the country and has strong ties to the Agency for Toxic Substances and Disease Registry. While her lab couldn't absolutely confirm the presence of a known heavy metal, she was quite suspicious the specimens we sent her contained either a previously unrecognized toxic heavy metal or a derivative of one or more of the known heavy metals."

"You can't be serious," Elias jumped in, as if he were talking to a poorly informed medical student.

"Don't I sound serious?" Jack asked him directly, which provoked a bit of a chuckle in the room.

Dr. Sam Arnold, a well-respected and perhaps the busiest cardiologist on staff, who tended to agree with Dr. Rutledge on most issues, signaled Connie.

"Go ahead, Sam."

"As one of the consulting cardiologists, I meticulously look at each of our patients' charts on a daily basis. I guess it's possible I could have overlooked it, but I don't recall seeing a report from Dr. Corsair's laboratory."

"You're correct, Sam," Kristin said. "Her report has not as yet been included in the medical record of any of the patients—that was my call."

"Your call, Kristin?" Rutledge asked in a voice dripping with indignation. "As the director of this group, I'd like to ask you how you convinced yourself that it was within your purview to censor the medical information that your fellow physicians have access to."

"I had no such intent. But for the record, the specimens were sent to her lab through normal channels as an official consultation. However, we just received the written report this morning, and I thought it would be better if we discussed the findings here at this meeting first. I assure you that, by this afternoon, Dr. Corsair's formal report will be on every patient's chart."

"Even so, Kristin. I'd say there's a clear conflict between what you think you're authorized to do and what we'd consider proper and ethical behavior."

"We'll just have to agree to disagree on your contention, but I think that's a conversation you and I can have in private at another time, Elias."

Kristin's expression remained unchanged. She reached forward and picked up a manila file folder she'd brought with her. She removed a stack of fifteen copies of Dr. Corsair's report and started them around the conference table. Kristin laid her disparaging eyes on Rutledge but stayed silent while the group read the report.

Sam said, "I don't know about the rest of you, but I'm clearly struck by the manner in which Dr. Corsair dictated her report. I find it more than a little vague. I understand she's in uncharted waters, but there's nothing definitive about her findings." Leisurely shaking his head, he drew his lips into a tight line. "In all honesty, I'd be very cautious about hanging our hats on this nebulous report."

"While I appreciate your observation, Sam, we should all bear in mind that Dr. Corsair is the director of one of the most prestigious laboratories in the country dealing with matters of heavy metal poisoning," Connie said, pausing to glance down at the report again. "I'd like Kristin to give us a review of her other reasons for believing these patients have been the victims of a toxic exposure and not an overwhelming viral infection."

For the next thirty minutes, Kristin reviewed all the clinical information that pointed to heavy metal poisoning in extreme detail. She stopped several times to answer questions from both the physicians and non-clinical people in attendance. She made it a point to emphasize the significance of Mees lines, the sudden onset of color blindness, and the presence of hiccups. At times, she yielded the floor to others who wished to offer their insights. On two occasions, Connie asked Jack and Madison for their opinions on a particular aspect of a patient's illness. Understanding their roles as consultants, they were direct and honest in their responses but ever cautious to do so in a collegial and professional manner. In the end, they made it clear the Marsh patients were likely to suffer a fatal outcome if their present treatment protocol wasn't urgently changed to focus on eradicating a deadly buildup of a heavy metal.

When they'd concluded, Connie shifted the conversation immediately to the arena of treatment.

"Because it would weigh heavily upon our decision, I think we'd all like to hear more details about the treatment you're recommending. I'm particularly interested in the types of complications our patients could encounter. Jack, Madison?"

"I'll take this," Madison said. "For many decades, chelation therapy has been the mainstay of treatment for heavy metal toxicity. The risks aren't overwhelming, but they're not insignificant either." She paused to give herself a chance to choose the best words to advise the group of the most dangerous and unorthodox aspect of their proposed treatment plan. "I'm afraid there's one other therapeutic intervention that we're going to have to give serious consideration to including in our treatment protocol," she said, lifting her eyes away from her notes to the group's inquisitive faces. "In view of how critically ill the patients are, we're proposing they all go on hemodialysis."

The murmur in the room that ensued was predictable.

"For how long?" Dr. Arch Britton asked.

"We haven't worked out the specific details yet, but we're guessing about five to seven days. And to be completely forthcoming, there's only limited evidence in the medical literature that dialysis can be relied upon to be helpful in patients who are critically ill with heavy metal poisoning."

Red-faced, Rutledge sprang to his feet, pushed his chair back, and glared at Connie.

"Are we to assume that you're in agreement with this ill-fated proposal?" he demanded to know.

"I'm taking everything I learn from this meeting under advisement. If you recall, the first thing I mentioned was that I'll advise everybody of my decision by the latest this evening."

"Why will you require extra time to make such an easy decision?"

Ignoring his question, Connie shifted her attention back to Madison. "Adding dialysis will also add risk, which begs the question: Just how imperative do you believe it is?"

"Jack and I are convinced that, if we exclude dialysis, it's highly unlikely chelation therapy, antioxidants, and Prussian blue alone will effect a cure. I'll be the first to admit, we don't have all the answers. But as we've mentioned, we may be dealing with a heavy metal that, until now, has been unknown to mainstream medicine, which would explain why currently available testing hasn't been able to isolate it."

"Two can play that game, Connie," Elias said.

"Excuse me?"

"Well, as long as we've now crossed over into pure theory, allow me to propose one. I'm sure we'd all agree that we know very little about this new strain of adenovirus that the Fort Detrick lab isolated. Perhaps this strain is more contagious and unpredictable than we've previously seen with other viruses. Maybe it's capable of infecting a small group of people who work in the same building." With a contemptuous grin, he added, "I say my theory's as plausible as Kristin's and should receive the same consideration."

Connie swung her gaze to Jack. "Assuming you're correct, any idea of how these folks got poisoned?"

He realized instantly that answering that question could open a large Pandora's box that could easily fuel Elias's contention the meeting was akin to the Theatre of the Absurd. Jack decided the smart move was to sidestep that minefield.

"We haven't been able to determine the portal of entry."

One of the attending physicians asked, "If we do decide to treat for heavy metal toxicity, would we have to discontinue the current antiviral therapy?"

Kristin fielded the question. "We checked with Infectious Diseases on that, and they said it would be safe to continue the medications the patients are currently on."

Connie took a few moments to gaze at the attendees. "I think we have a very accurate picture of the challenges we're facing with these patients. Are there any other questions?" When nobody in the room responded, she said, "We have ten voting physicians present. By a show of hands, how many believe we should offer the families heavy metal toxicity therapy, which will include a short course of dialysis?" There was a moderate amount of hesitancy, but in the end, eight of the doctors indicated the affirmative.

Aaron Steele asked, "You mentioned at the beginning of the meeting that you'd make a decision by this evening. Is that still your intention?"

"Actually, I'm comfortable giving you my decision right now. We've already lost two patients to this illness. From the information I've been able to gather from several sources, we're on the cusp of losing two more. To me, this is a simple matter of risk versus consequences. I'm convinced that if we don't change course we'll lose every one of these patients. If they are suffering from heavy metal poisoning and we don't try to do something about it, we'll be making a tragic mistake. If we can continue the antiviral therapy, I see no reason we can't carefully explain the risks, complications, and possible alternatives of our proposed plan of treatment to the family members and allow them to decide."

"With all due respect, Connie, I think that's a very ill-advised decision," Rutledge stated with a mixture of authority and frustration.

"Your objection to my decision is noted."

"I'm the leader of the physician task group, yet you dismiss my opinions as irrelevant," Rutledge told her, giving his chair a shove backward and rising to his feet.

"I have every respect for your opinions, Elias. I just don't happen to agree with you on this particular issue." Without responding, he stormed out of the conference room. Ignoring his petulant behavior, Connie concluded her remarks to the group. "Unless there are any other questions, I thank everybody present for taking the time to attend this meeting. Please clear your schedules for this afternoon so we can meet to begin formulating a specific treatment plan." She turned and faced Kristin. "For those families who elect to proceed, when will you be ready to begin?"

"All the patients will require a special intravenous catheter to undergo dialysis. With the assistance of our interventional radiologists and surgeons, I'm hopeful we can them placed today and begin dialysis as early as tonight. As far as the chelation and Prussian blue therapy are concerned, as long as we have the meds in house, we can begin at any time we choose."

"Which brings me to my next request," Connie said. "I'd like the task group to meet again as soon as possible, break down into smaller groups, and create a detailed treatment plan. I realize we're under the gun, but we can't lose sight of the fact that it's absolutely imperative that we avoid any mistakes in our care of these patients. The last thing we need is to commit an egregious medical error."

Chapter 52

As Connie had requested, at noon, the members of the task group met and broke down into three smaller subgroups, each to address a specific aspect of treating heavy metal poisoning. When their individual meetings were finished, the plan was for the subgroups to join together, share their ideas, and finalize a detailed protocol to be used to treat the Marsh patients. By two o'clock, the subgroups had adjourned and were ready to bring their recommendations to the combined meeting.

Waiting for it to begin, Jack and Madison were talking to Kristin in the hall when Connie walked up and joined them. If she were trying to disguise her dismay, the disenchanted look on her face wasn't helping.

"We have a bit of a problem," she wasted no time telling them. "I assume Dr. Rutledge didn't participate in any of the subgroup meetings."

"He was supposed to be in the dialysis group with me, but he never showed," Kristin said. "I assumed he got tied up with a patient problem."

"I don't think so. An hour ago, he knocked on my office door in a rather indecent mood. I'll skip all the ranting and raving and just cut to the chase. He resigned from the task group and made a number of not-so-lightly veiled threats to report our irresponsible, unethical, and malfeasant treatment of the Marsh patients."

"To whom?" Kristin inquired.

"He wasn't specific, but I'm guessing to anybody who'd be inclined to listen to him." The three of them didn't utter a word as they watched Connie sadly shake her head. She leveled her eyes on Kristin. "So, first things first. Since Elias has seen fit to resign, I'd appreciate it if you'd once again take charge of the task group."

"I'd be pleased to, but I'm not sure Aaron Steele will be too happy about it."

"When I want Mr. Steele's opinion regarding medical matters, I'll ask for it. In the first place, I don't work for him, and in the second, I consider this a patient care crisis, wholly in the hands of the physicians. If anybody wants to grumble about my decision, they know where to find me." Connie pushed a determined look to her face. As she did, Kristin gave her a thumbs-up in support of her bravado. "So may I assume we're all reading from the same playbook?"

"Absolutely," Kristin assured her.

The way Connie was standing with her arms straight down at her sides and her sudden silence gave Madison reason to suspect there was something else on her mind. It didn't take long for her suspicion to be confirmed.

"The other matter I want to mention it that, before Elias stormed into my office, I met with Arch Britton and the nursing leadership. There seems to be major concern that the patients are deteriorating so rapidly that there is no treatment that will turn things around."

"They may be right, but hopefully, we'll be able to change their minds," Jack said. "But in spite of everything we try, there's still a chance we could lose every one of them. Unfortunately, I don't think that possibility justifies standing idly by and letting nature take its course."

"The only reason I mention it is to make sure that whatever treatment plan the group decides upon, make sure you roll it out as quickly and as safely as possible. And most importantly, let's keep the lines of communication open with the nurses and the other staff."

Madison said, "Since dialysis will probably turn out to be the most important part of our treatment protocol, we're going to recommend CRRT over standard dialysis."

"You'll have to excuse me, but my nephrology's a little rusty. What's CRRT?"

"Continuous renal replacement therapy. We'd keep the patients on dialysis twenty-four hours a day," Madison answered. "After three days, when we change the circuit, we can make a determination whether to continue or not."

"Kayla Shireman's a member of the task group and, as I'm sure you know, an outstanding nephrologist," Kristin said. "She's also the codirector of our dialysis program and will supervise the CRRT. As soon as we give her the word, she'll be ready to start."

"And the medications you'll be using?" Connie inquired.

Jack answered, "We'll select the specific chelating agents and the schedule we'll use to administer them at the meeting. We'll also add the antioxidants and vitamins that are typically used in treating heavy metal toxicity."

"The chelation meds and dialysis schedule for each patient may vary a little depending on his or her condition," Madison added. "We'll need to review that twice a day at least."

"It looks like most of the patients will have their dialysis catheters in by early this evening. So as we discussed earlier, it may be a good idea to push for beginning dialysis tonight," Jack said. "I know it's a little unusual to initiate major treatments at night, but this is one of those situations where every hour we save could make a difference."

"I think Jack's suggestion's right on point," Madison said.

"I'll make sure I make the recommendation at the meeting," Kristin said. "I'm sure Kayla will have no objections. As soon as the meeting's over, we'll advise the families of our plan."

"I know all the consents are signed, but I suspect we'll still get some additional pretty tough questions," Connie said.

"We'll be ready," Kristin assured her. "Are you planning on attending the meeting?"

"You're darn right I am," she answered as an undeniable look of determination came to rest on her face.

THE COMBINED meeting of the subgroups lasted two hours and was extremely productive. The cooperative spirit in the room was praiseworthy. The therapy document that the group created was a detailed timeline of the rollout and the precise steps to be followed on each successive day.

Following the meeting, all of the families were again invited to discuss the risks and alternatives to the proposed therapy plan and any additional concerns they had. None of them had a change of heart, and each of the nine patients was scheduled to participate in a five phase dialysis and chelation treatment protocol.

By five o'clock the next afternoon, every one of them had completed **PHASE I**.

Part IV

Chapter 53

PHASE II

Seated in the hotel restaurant for the past forty minutes, Jack and Madison shared the quietest meal either of them could recall. The treatment protocol had been rolled out seamlessly, and they were encouraged by how well the patients were tolerating the dialysis and the medications. There had been some minor complications, but when considering the patients' critical condition and the scope of the therapy, a few small setbacks were to be expected. Unfortunately, the encouraging news was greatly diminished by the stark reality that none of the patients were showing any signs of improvement.

They arrived at the hospital at a few minutes before eight. While Madison began reviewing the latest clinical information on the patients, Jack decided to check on Nicole. He made his way toward her room with a bit of trepidation, wondering what would await him on the other side of her door. It had become his custom to call her nurse each morning before breakfast, but on this particular morning he hadn't.

The moment he entered the room, his worst nightmare came true. Arch Britton and two nurses intently hovered over Nicole.

From the looks on their faces, it wasn't hard to connect the dots. Jack relocated his gaze to the monitors. Nicole's pulse rate was too rapid, and her blood pressure was teetering on dangerously low. Her face was flushed.

Before Jack could say anything, Arch looked up.

"I'm afraid we have a problem, Jack. It looks like she's having a severe allergic reaction to one of the chelating agents. I'm guessing it was the deferiprone. Her hives, wheezing, and facial swelling are pretty typical of anaphylaxis. We've already given her epi. I'm going to hold off on antihistamines and steroids until we see how she responds to our first line treatment."

"How bad's her respiratory status?"

"She's tight and definitely working harder to breath, but for now her oxygen saturation's okay. We worked pretty damn hard to get her off the vent, which means I'm going to do everything I can not to put her back on."

"What about stopping the dialysis?"

"I spoke with Kayla. She's on her way over now to take a look, but for now she wants to keep it going."

Jack was trying to remain optimistic, but it was a struggle. At that moment, Madison came through the door.

She took one look around and asked, "What's going on?"

"It looks like Nicole's had anaphylactic reaction to one of the chelation meds. Arch thinks it's the deferiprone."

After looking at the monitors, Madison took a few steps closer to the bed.

"I've got this, Jack" Arch said, tossing a concerned glance at Madison. "I'm going to stay here with Nicole, so if you guys want to continue rounds, go ahead. I'll come get you if things go south." From the strain in Arch's voice, Madison guessed they were thinking the same thing—Jack's anxiety level was approaching the red line and the last thing he needed was to watch Nicole fight her way through another crisis.

.   .   .

"THAT SOUNDS LIKE A GOOD IDEA, JACK," Madison said placing her hand on his forearm. She realized he was aware of what she was doing, but as she expected, he didn't voice any objections. Not wasting any time, she thanked Arch with a quick nod, and ushered Jack out of the room.

For the next couple of hours, they made rounds on the remaining eight patients. Jack did his best to focus on the task at hand but he was distracted by his concern for Nicole. He had always been a strong believer in the medical wisdom that patients generally tolerate intense therapy regimens— but what they don't tolerate well are complications. He was beyond alarmed that her unexpected anaphylactic reaction might be enough to push her over the edge and negate any chance she had to recover.

They decided to take a few minutes and go to the physicians' lounge and grab a cup of coffee.

"So far, I'd say our treatment protocol has been ineffective," he said flatly.

"I agree, but it's a little early to think about waving the white flag."

"I know."

"I have an idea. Why don't we track down Anise and see if she can meet us for lunch?"

"I spoke with her earlier. She's got a pretty busy day at school. I don't think she'll be able to. She's not planning on coming to the hospital until tonight."

"Hopefully by then, she'll be doing a lot better," Madison said.

"I hope so too. I think I'll go back and check on her now."

"It's only been a couple of hours, Jack," she reminded him.

"I know, but it's possible she could have responded favorably fairly quickly. I won't be long."

Madison was just about to offer to accompany him, but she suddenly thought better of the idea and decided it might be better if he went alone. She watched with trepidation as he walked down the hall, wondering what she could do to boost his spirits a little. If there was something, it certainly didn't spring to her mind.

Chapter 54

PHASE III

With Tess alongside her, Anise walked across Georgetown Infirmary's lobby. Griffin, the escort Mike had sent with Tess, trailed a few steps behind them. Before they checked in at the welcome center, Tess suggested he wait for them in the lobby. To everyone's relief, since she'd arrived, Anise had had no further concerns regarding her security.

After checking in at the welcome center, they went straight up to the fourth floor to visit Nicole. It had taken eleven hours of intensive therapy, but much to the delight and relief of those caring for her, she had made it through her major allergic episode with no apparent adverse consequences.

Similar to Nicole, the other eight patients were holding their own. But to their caregivers' dismay, none were showing any meaningful signs of improvement. The one encouraging development that heralded the possibility of a favorable outcome was that all but two of the patients had been taken off the ventilator and were breathing on their own without any difficulty. Unfortunately, they were still in a neurologically impaired state and not responsive.

Having been able to adopt the time-honored approach of hoping for the best but preparing for the worst, Anise had reached a glum but steady state.

It was a few minutes before seven a.m. when Anise and Tess walked into Nicole's room. Her nurse, Miranda, was sitting in front of the computer making entries into the nursing notes section of Nicole's electronic medical record. During the first phase of treatment Jack had taken the time to carefully explain the process of dialysis to Anise, so the sight of the machine wouldn't shock her.

"Good morning to you both," Miranda said, walking over and taking Anise's hands in hers. "How are you doing?"

"Maybe a little."

"Isn't this a little early for you? I'm used to seeing you at the end of my shift."

"I have a lot of stuff to do at school today, so I thought I'd come in early." As she always did, she relocated one of the chairs to the head of the bed and sat down. Tess quietly moved to the other side of the room to allow Anise some alone time with Nicole. "Did Mom have a good night?" she asked Miranda.

"I'd say she's stable. Your father and the team haven't made rounds yet, but I'm expecting them any time now."

Anise had reached a point where she could get a pretty good idea of her mom's condition from simply looking at her complexion and studying her eyes, especially how often she blinked. Warning herself to be objective, Anise studied her for a few seconds longer than usual because she was convinced that some color and animation had returned to her face. She was also surprised to see her right arm and hand weren't tucked under the covers as they usually were. When she looked back at her mom's face, she immediately jumped up from her chair. At the same moment, she covered her mouth, and her eyes began to tear up.

"Miranda, can you please come over here for a sec?"

"Sure," she said, moving to Anise's side.

"Look at Mom's eyes. I swear she just blinked them a couple of times, and then held them open for a few moments. After she closed them for a couple of seconds, she did the same thing again. I…I may be losing my mind, but I think she recognized me."

"A few of the patients have been opening their eyes more frequently for the last twenty-four hours. It's an encouraging sign, but the doctors have warned us not to read too much into it."

"The doctors may be wrong," Anise said, keeping her eyes glued on her mother's face. A brief period of time passed without her repeating the eye movement. Just as Anise was about to give up, she saw her raise her hand ever so slightly. She then moved it slowly toward the center of the bed, and then laid it on her tummy. Anise instantly looked at Miranda, taking note of the astonished look on her face. She knew she'd seen the same thing she did. Anise's face lit up like the glow of a sunrise.

"That's the most purposeful movement I've seen your mom make since we started treatment," Miranda said with an elated grin and a slight hitch in her voice.

Tess moved to the bedside, and the three of them stood shoulder to shoulder in expectant silence with their eyes glued on Nicole. After a few seconds, she rolled her head a few inches to the right, opened her eyes, and looked at them with undeniable purpose. Anise feared she was hallucinating, but she could have sworn the corners of her mother's mouth curled ever so slightly into the beginnings of a smile.

"My god," Miranda uttered in just above a whisper, as she brought her fingertips to her lips. "I'm going to find the team," she announced, as she turned and hurried toward the door.

Anise felt the accelerated contractions of her heart from the visceral an adrenaline rush. Reaching down, she took her mom's hand in hers. At first it was entirely flaccid, but a few moments later she felt her mom's frail attempt to squeeze it. She brought her lips to within a few inches of her mom's ear.

"Can you hear me, Mom?" There was no answer. "Just squeeze my hand a little if you're able to hear me." Still nothing. Her eyes flashed to the door, wondering when Miranda would return with her dad. Confused and unable to hold a clear thought in her head, Anise repeated her request. By the way her mom's eyes moved over her face, she was sure it was anything but a random look. She renewed her question, "Can you hear me, Mom?"

Nicole's lips quivered briefly and then came together in a line. Her chin then inched downward in what Anise believed was as an attempt to nod.

All of a sudden, she felt her mom's hand squeeze hers. Consumed with joy, she felt her own hands trembling. She and Tess exchanged a joyous look and they began to sob. It was at that moment that Miranda came through the door with Jack, Madison, and Kristin right behind her. They all hastened to the bedside.

Jack checked the cardiac monitor. Nicole's vital signs and oxygen level were right on the money. His eyes came to rest on her face. The smile he knew so well appeared on her face. Everybody in the room saw it prompting Anise to pull them all into a mighty hug.

Anise quickly returned to her chair, sat down, and again placed her lips close to her mother's ear.

"Hey, Mom. You're going to be okay. Dad's here. So are Madison and Aunt Tess."

Nicole whispered, "Hi, Shortstuff." It was all she could manage.

"Thank god," Tess whispered.

"Looks like somebody's feeling better," Madison said, her smile showing her unique understanding of what it felt like to begin to recover from a life-threatening illness.

It looked to Miranda as if Nicole was trying to mouth something. She stepped forward and dropped down to place her ear a few inches from Nicole's lips.

A blissful smile illuminated Miranda's face.

"It seems our patient would like some cranberry juice. Any problem with that, Doctors?"

"By all means," Kristin said, accompanied with a fist pump. Madison smiled inwardly at her uncharacteristic public display of emotion.

Tess gave Jack another hug. "I guess you and Madison can add Nicole's name to those of us who owe our lives to you two."

Chapter 55

PHASE V

It was two days later, and the pure elation that filled the halls of the intermediate care unit of the Georgetown Infirmary was still palpable. Phases four and five of chelation therapy and dialysis had now been completed, with the vast majority of the neurologic symptoms having completely resolved. It was one of the most rapid recoveries from a critical illness that Jack and Madison had ever witnessed. The only exception was John Winkler, whose neurologic function was somewhat slower in returning than the other patients.

It was a few minutes after six in the evening when Jack and Madison were finishing up rounds. By this point, visiting the patients was becoming more of a social activity than a medical necessity.

"We haven't seen Lori yet," Madison reminded him.

"I assumed you intentionally left her for last."

"As long as nobody else is listening, I'll admit she's kind of my favorite. I've gotten to know Gretchen pretty well. She's quite an individual."

"The baby's still doing well?"

"She'll need to be considered high risk and monitored carefully until she's born, but under the circumstances, I'd say she's doing great."

They reached Lori's room. Madison tapped a couple of times on the sliding glass door, and they entered. She was pleased to see Lori was out of bed and sitting in a lounger. Gretchen was standing behind her massaging her shoulders.

"Somebody looks like they're almost ready to go home," Madison said as she crossed the room.

"The rumor is we're out of here either tomorrow or the day after," Gretchen said, kissing Lori on the cheek and then reaching around and gingerly patting her tummy for good luck.

Lori stretched her hands high above her head. "I still feel pretty washed out, but it's nice to rejoin the human race. I'm ready to go home—that's for sure."

"We've been over your chart, and I must say it looks every bit as good as you do," Madison said. "How's your appetite?"

"I've been on a regular diet since yesterday. For a hospital, this place has a pretty good chef."

"As evidenced by the fact that she's eating like a Viking," Gretchen said. "She's also renewed her addiction to reading books so I assume her brain's back to working normally. She must have a thousand books downloaded on her tablet, and she's picked up right where she left off when she got sick."

"How's your eyesight? Are you able to read okay?" Jack asked.

"No problem at all. I even remember the plot of my latest book."

"She's the most avid reader I've ever seen."

"I think you already mentioned that, Gretch. You'll have to excuse my wife. She tends to exaggerate to extreme."

"Really? If it hadn't been for the book club you and John Winkler started, you wouldn't have survived Covid."

"I belong to a book club too," Madison said. "I love it. Is yours still going on?"

"It was until about a week ago, but I'm sure we'll get it fired up again after we're all discharged."

Jack and Madison shared an intrigued look.

"How many of the patients are Marsh employees?" Madison asked.

"All of them, I think. When we started the club, we got up to about thirty-five members. But about six months ago, some of us got interested in writing, and we carved out a much smaller group so we could exchange what we'd written and critique each other's work."

"How often were you guys meeting?" Madison asked.

"We were all working from home at the time, so I'd say two or three times a week. John Winkler's wife, Suzy, stopped in earlier to see how I was doing. She mentioned some of the other Marsh employees from our writing group had also been admitted. Are you both readers?"

"Dr. Wyatt loves historical fiction, but I lean more toward narrative nonfiction."

"If you're ever interested in joining another club, just let me know. We'd love to have you both. It would be nice to have some members who don't work at Marsh."

"Thanks, we may take you up on that," she said.

"I'll put you on our email list. It'll give you an idea of the types of books we discuss."

"I'd love to take a look at it. Does your smaller group have a separate email chain?"

"We do, and I can add you and Dr. Wyatt to that chain as well if you'd like. Have you written anything you'd like to submit?"

"I'm afraid not, but it's something I've thought about trying for a long time."

"You should give it a shot. In the beginning, it's kind of hard letting other people read your work. It's sort of like singing in public for the first time. But once you break the ice, it's a lot of fun."

"Does everybody in the group feel that way?"

"I think so...except maybe for John. He can be a wet blanket sometimes. He once told us that asking your friends for their opinion on your writing is like asking your mother if you're good looking."

"Interesting analogy," Jack said with a grin.

"If you leave me your email address, I'll forward our latest emails from both groups."

Jack and Madison spent the next few minutes talking more to Lori about how she was feeling and her plans once she was discharged. Jack did a cursory neurologic exam, and as he'd expected, he found nothing that concerned him.

"Will you be in to see us tomorrow?" Gretchen asked.

"We should be making rounds at about this same time."

Gretchen walked them to the door. "She's doing great," she whispered. "I'm starting to run out of ways to thank you two."

The moment they stepped into the hall, Jack turned to Madison. "I know what you're thinking, and it's probably just a coincidence."

"Maybe, but it's too much of a coincidence to simply dismiss it out of hand. Anyway, it shouldn't be hard to check."

"Even if your hunch is right and all eleven Marsh patients were part of the book club, I'm not sure it would mean anything."

"I guess as soon as we find that out for sure one way or the other, we'll be able to talk about it."

They continued down the hall. Jack said, "I noticed you've been coughing a little the past couple of days—are you feeling okay?"

"I'm fine, Jack."

"Did you check in with Kay or one of your other hematologists?"

"I didn't think it was necessary—not yet anyway." He didn't say anything more, prompting Madison to take note of the uneasy look on his face. "If it continues for another couple of days, I'll give Kay a call." She held up a hand and added, "I promise." She was about to remind him how often they were having this same conversation, but after another few moments of thought, she dismissed the idea.

"Fair enough."

"Why don't we see the rest of these folks and then track down Kristin? It's about time we spoke to her about signing off...don't you think?"

"I do. Nicole should be going home tomorrow. I'm sure Anise

will want to postpone the college tour for a while to be with her," Jack said, watching Madison agree with a nod.

An hour later, they were done with what they guessed might be their last chart review. Madison reached for her phone and checked her inbox. As promised, Lori had sent her two emails. After studying them briefly, her quintessential knowing smile appeared on her face. She handed Jack the phone.

"It looks like the aspiring writers group was made up of our eleven patients," she said, setting her searching eyes on him.

"You have the information you were after."

"It certainly poses an interesting question as to how a virtual writing group could all come down with same illness within a few days of each other," Madison said. "The other matter worth considering is, if we don't know how or why these folks suffered the toxic exposure in the first place, how do we know it won't happen again?"

"We don't. But if it does, the physicians here should be able to handle the problem. Don't you think?"

"Actually, I don't," she said flatly. "Because of the success of the treatment plan, everybody's pretty much in agreement that the patients were all victims of a large dose of an unidentifiable heavy metal." She stopped and placed her hand on his arm, prompting him to stop as well. "Don't you find it just a tad on the strange side that not a single doctor or administrator at this hospital has raised the possibility that just maybe these patients were intentionally poisoned?"

"I do, but then, when I consider the obvious follow-up question, it no longer seems like much of a mystery."

"What follow-up question?" he asked.

"Why would anybody want to poison eleven random employees — and even if that were the case, wouldn't it be a matter best left for the authorities to deal with?"

Chapter 56

Everett Warren wasn't in the least bit surprised when he received a call from Brubaker to set up a meeting as soon as possible. He assumed the reason was to inform him that, because matters involving the Marsh patients had come to an unsatisfactory conclusion, a cooling-off period was called for before they would readdress the problem.

It was ten minutes past three on a temperate fall day when Claude turned the Maybach limousine east on Independence Avenue. When he reached the spot where the West Potomac Park was directly across from the Korean Soldiers War Memorial, he pulled over to the curb. Claude immediately exited the limousine and opened the door for Brubaker who settled into the same seat he'd occupied the first time they met.

This time, however, he didn't waste any time engaging in gratuitous pleasantries.

"Let's not spin our wheels dwelling on what went wrong and assigning blame. We need to focus on how we'll be moving forward."

Warren nodded. "The matter of the patients' recovery is still drawing a lot of attention. I'm not suggesting we abandon the problem, but it might be in our best interests to let all the excitement pass for a month or so before we decide what to do next."

"Everything's a matter of perspective and choices, and not to sound too cliché, every problem has a solution." Exhaling a near bottomless breath, Brubaker added, "We don't have months to deal with this problem, nor the option to simply pick up our ball and go home with our tails between our legs."

"I was just trying to—"

"Whatever you're going to say is a moot point and not worth discussing because I don't have the luxury of modifying my instruction," Brubaker told him curtly.

Warren considered trying to clarify his suggestion, but when he realized he wouldn't be taken seriously, he dismissed the idea in favor of raising a new concern. "We can't overlook Ed Terry from the Defense Contract Management Agency."

"If my memory serves me correctly, he was tragically killed in a mugging while he was out walking his dog."

"I'm referring to whatever records he may have left behind from his meeting with Oren Severin regarding John Winkler's report."

"Let's just say that was included in our original assessment, and as far as the existence of any credible documentation, that meeting never took place," Brubaker said. "Now, I suggest we move on. As I've already mentioned, time remains a critical factor."

"Let's not forget about John Winkler. We need to deal with him before he gets another bright idea to disclose what he thinks he knows."

"Based on his current neurologic condition, I don't think that's a pressing issue. We have some time to a figure out the best way of handling that situation," Brubaker said before changing directions. "That leaves the other eight Marsh patients who could have a sudden brainstorm and create a major problem for us. Even though we hoped it wouldn't, the story has captured the public's attention. But as is true with most intriguing events, it'll soon be last week's news. As far as we know, everybody's ecstatic about the patients' recoveries, and nobody's raised the possibility that they were the victims of anything nefarious. We need that to continue, because if it doesn't, our situation could rapidly become unsustainable."

"It's possible that embarrassing or damaging information could already be out there and we're simply not aware of it."

"That's simply a chance we'll have to take," Brubaker didn't hesitate to tell him. "The reason I requested this meeting is to leave you with the following instructions: From your perspective, nothing has changed. Do not for any reason take matters into your own hands, and you're to remain tight-lipped until you hear from me again. Is that understood?"

"Yes."

"Obviously, our goal is to come up with a new solution that will have the same endpoint."

Warren gazed out the window for a few moments. "Are you recommending a change in your choice of freelancers?"

"I don't think that'll be necessary, but everything's up for consideration."

As was the case the first time they'd met, Warren found himself uncharacteristically intimidated by Brubaker. He could feel droplets of perspiration forming on the back of his neck. He opened the refrigerator and removed a short bottle of flavored sparkling water. "What would you like me to do?"

"The only other thing you need to do is let me off at the next corner."

The moment Brubaker was out of the limousine, Warren took a long swallow of water. He was experienced enough to recognize a situation that provided no wiggle room. He'd hoped he'd be able to find a way to lengthen the fuse on the problem, but that obviously didn't happen.

He let his head fall back and closed his eyes, resolving himself to the reality that his best course of action was to silently fall in line, maintain a low profile, and do exactly what he was told.

Chapter 57

It had been a week since the last Marsh patient had been declared well and discharged from the hospital. Nicole's full recovery was among the fastest of the patients. From the time she got home, she'd been working a few hours a day with no problems. In the last day or so, she'd become anxious to resume her full-time schedule at Marsh.

Everett Warren had arranged a formal dinner, inviting the organization's key leadership and the doctors who'd served on the task group to attend. The dinner was scheduled for six p.m. and included an elaborate menu that would have duly impressed anybody, irrespective of how many elegantly catered high-end dinners they'd attended. Having just come through a major corporate crisis, the mood in the room was understandably jovial. Prior to dinner, the attendees engaged in friendly conversations, sampled a wide variety of hors d'oeuvres, and enjoyed a fully stocked bar.

With a broad smile, Warren raised his hand. "If everybody will find their seat, we can dispense with the preliminaries and enjoy our dinner." He waited a few moments while everyone settled in at one of the tables before continuing. "Seven days ago marked a huge red-letter day in the history of Marsh Technologies. Our final patient suffering from a terrible illness was discharged home to their loving family. Unfortunately, we lost two valued colleagues. I don't believe that's something any of us will ever get over." Bowing his head he paused for a few seconds before going on, "As the chairman of the board, it's my great honor to thank everybody here this evening. You all played a vital role in successfully dealing with one of the most difficult challenges our great organization has ever faced. What we accomplished together was the perfect union of a great medical team and a corporate leadership who embraces its relationship with every employee, not just in words, but in action. I'm so damn proud of everybody, I hardly know how to express myself." He raised a finger in a way that seemed to indicate a change of heart. "It was my intention not to thank anybody individually tonight, but I've changed my mind." He turned, faced Jack and Madison, and raised his glass. "A special toast of gratitude to Drs. Shaw and Wyatt. We will remain eternally grateful for the critical part each of you played in this medical miracle." With the exception of Elias Rutledge, the room filled with enthusiastic applause as they toasted Madison and Jack. "And now, I'd like to yield the podium to Kasey Silverstrom, our director of human resources, who has come up with another one of her brilliant ideas that she and I are busting at the seams to share with you."

A twenty-year employee and a woman of style, grace, and polish, Kasey came to her feet.

"Warren, I'm sure I speak for all of us when I thank you for your continued inspired leadership and for generously signing off on this very special and pricey expression of appreciation I proposed to you." When the laughter died down, she continued. "Our remarkable medical team informs me that, in the next week or so, they anticipate clearing our special nine employees to embark on a blue-sky holiday that we hope they'll never forget." A proud grin came to her face as she went on. "We are currently arranging for them, along with their guests, to be flown to San Juan on one of our company jets. After three days in Puerto Rico, they will set sail on a week-long luxurious cruise on a private yacht." The room once again filled with applause and the murmur of conversation. "I thank Warren again and invite you all to enjoy the rest of the evening."

The remainder of the night's celebration was filled with great food, considerable back-patting, an endless choice of libations, and lighthearted conversation. The atmosphere was one of optimism for the company's continued success. Jack and Madison were a little overwhelmed by the opulence. When Warren made his final comments and the evening came to its conclusion, they stopped to talk to Kristin on their way out.

"I can't say I've attended a lot of dinners like that," Madison said.

"There was quite a bit of pomp and circumstance," Kristin answered in a voice laced with sarcasm as Elias approached. He wasted no time sharing his take on the outcome with them.

"It's hard to know how much of this fortunate outcome was nothing more than pure luck."

Kristin's eyes narrowed. "Excuse me?"

"We never had one shred of hard scientific evidence that our patients suffered a dangerous exposure to a heavy metal. Did it ever occur to the three of you that perhaps we had the correct diagnosis from day one, and these folks simply recovered on their own?" For Jack's part, he saw no reason to respond. He suspected Kristin felt the same, and he prayed Madison did as well. Elias added with a haughty shrug, "I didn't think you'd choose to answer the question. It's just possible you subjected nine critically ill patients to a dangerous course of hemodialysis and medications they never needed." He started to walk away. "If you'll excuse me, I have to get back to the hospital. I have a patient to see."

They waited until he was out of earshot.

"Don't even bother. His comments don't warrant a response," Kristin said. "So when are you guys taking Anise on the college tour?"

"She'd like to stay with Nicole a while longer. We haven't decided yet if we'll stay in DC for a while longer or head back to Columbus and return when we have a final date for the trip."

"Let me know when you finalize your plans. There's that matter of a fancy dinner out I still owe you."

"We wouldn't miss it for the world," he said.

Jack and Madison exited the building. While they were waiting for the van to be brought around, she said, "Maybe it's me, but from the joyous atmosphere this evening, it's hard to believe that anybody in the room tonight except you, me, and Kristin has even the slightest interest in trying to figure out how these folks got exposed to a toxic dose of a heavy metal."

"The last I heard, Marsh hired the most prestigious firm in the US to do a thorough evaluation of the corporate headquarters to make sure they're compliant with OSHA's heavy metal guidelines and requirements."

Madison looked at him through unconvinced eyes. "A nice gesture on their part, but if that investigation turns up anything, I'll be astounded."

Chapter 58

As soon as Erik finished responding to his last email of the day, he grabbed his sport coat, said a quick bye to his staff, and headed for the elevator. It was only five p.m., which made it likely, even with the evening traffic, that he'd be home by six—a welcome exception to what he was accustomed to. He was crossing the lobby when he caught sight of a familiar figure. He sighed on the inside as his upbeat mood was replaced by an immediate tailspin.

"How are you, Erik?" Regan asked.

"I'm okay, but I am a little surprised to see you."

"And why's that?"

"Because I never expected to see you again."

"Never's a long time. May I walk with you to your parking lot?"

"It's a free country."

"I'm not sure everybody would agree with that, but I'll tag along anyway. If my understanding's correct regarding the Marsh patients, the prevailing opinion is that, while the illness was an enigma, nobody knows how they contracted it."

"I don't know, but I'm guessing your information is almost certainly more current than mine."

"It seems the main focus of attention is on the brilliant treatment provided by the Georgetown Infirmary medical staff and their invited consultants from Ohio."

"I think it's only natural that the medical team would be proud of what they accomplished," he said, picking up his pace as they exited the building and headed toward the parking lot. "I'll exclude the possibility that you just happened to be loitering in our lobby when you saw me step off the elevator. Why don't you tell me what's on your mind?"

"You're a little grumpy this afternoon. I'm here as a courtesy to you."

"That's a little hard to believe, but I'm listening."

"I understand you weren't briefed on the key details of what was going on. But I assume you were aware that we were working our tails off trying to correct a very delicate problem."

"You still haven't told me what you're doing here."

"I just wanted to let you know the matter of the Marsh patients is closed," she told him. "We have no further interest in your company's problems."

"I'll assume that's good news, but two of our employees are dead. Whom should their families see about that?"

"I admit to nothing, and I'm not here as a psychiatrist," she made clear. "As I said, I'm here merely as a courtesy to bring you up to speed on things."

"A courtesy? That's an interesting word choice. And what inspired this miraculous display of good manners and forthrightness?"

"You're shooting the messenger, Erik. Your guess is as good as mine. Similar to you, I don't give a hoot in hell what their reasons are. The important thing is that what I'm telling you is absolute and permanent. Have a nice evening."

She stopped, turned, and started back in the opposite direction. Erik never broke stride, and neither of them thought to give the other a final glance.

As he entered the parking lot, he couldn't help but wonder why

Regan had gone out of her way to ambush him. He hardly knew her, but he had the impression that there was a method to her madness in most things she said and did.

Part V

Chapter 59

TWO WEEKS LATER

Jack and Madison arrived back in DC on the first non-stop of the day out of Columbus. Their plan was to check into their hotel, spend a leisurely day sightseeing before meeting Anise for dinner to go over their final plans for her college tour.

Jack had just gotten off the phone with Anise when Madison walked into the room.

"How's everything? Are we all set?"

"Nicole's doing very well and Anise is comfortable about leaving her for a few days. She's all set to meet us for dinner tonight and get an early start in the morning."

"Great, so what's on our agenda for today?" Madison asked.

"Well, if you can find a way to kill an hour or so, I'm going to have a final look at a manuscript I promised to review. It should take me about an hour. As soon as I'm done, I'm all yours."

"Pinky swear?" she teased, waiting for Jack to wrap his little finger around hers.

"Absolutely."

"As soon as you're ready, how about going for a run and then heading over to H Street

for some Chinese food?"

Jack gave her a thumbs-up and headed over to the desk.

While he was getting to work, Madison flopped down into the corner of the couch and began checking her emails. While she was searching for the one she'd received from an old college friend, she came across Lori's email that included the submissions from the members of the writing group. Once Madison had determined that everybody in the group had been admitted to the Infirmary with heavy metal poisoning, reading the submissions didn't seem very important and it quickly slipped her mind.

Having some time to spare while she waited for Jack, her curiosity now got the best of her, and she decided to take a look at a few of them. When she did, she found herself more impressed than she suspected she would be. The fourth one she opened was John Winkler's. It didn't take her long to see it was the first few chapters and a plot synopsis of a novel, leaving her intrigued enough to have a closer look at it.

The next time she lifted her eyes from the text was when she'd finished reading every word of it. She was still thinking about John's work when Jack got up from the desk.

"You're not dressed," he said. "Are you still interested in going for a run?" When she didn't respond, he strolled over to her and immediately took note of the troubled look on her face. "What's going on?"

"I think you should read this."

"What is it?"

"It's John Winkler's submission to the writing group that Lori told us about. It's the first few chapters and a synopsis of a novel he claimed he was working on."

"Claimed he was working on?"

"I'm not so sure. That's why I want you to read it."

"Now?" he asked, seeing the uneasiness in her eyes.

"Yeah, and while you do, I'll go for that run."

"Without me? I thought we were going to do that together."

"I'm not sure we'll have time for a recreational activity after you read it, and I could use the exercise."

"I see...I think."

———

AN HOUR LATER, Madison opened the door to their hotel suite. Jack was at the desk with his eyes fixed on her laptop's screen, busily scribbling away on one of the hotel's notepads.

"What do you think?" she asked him, kicking off her running shoes.

"I share your uncertainty that John meant it purely as the work of a fledgling novelist."

"My thoughts exactly. What next?"

"I was just asking myself the same question. I don't think ignoring it is an option. Who do you think we should call?"

"I'd say Kristin. It should be her call on how to take this new...new wrinkle up the chain of command."

"I'm not sure I agree with that."

"Why?"

"Because I'm not certain how far up the chain of command she'll get before somebody harpoons it," he stated. "I'm also concerned that, before it's over, Kristin will turn out to be the proverbial rabbit sitting around a table with five coyotes trying to decide what they're going to have for lunch." He slowly closed the lid of Madison's laptop. "I think we should call Special Agent Banks, and I think we should do it right now."

She pinched her lips together and nodded. "Okay."

Jack reached for his phone and held it up. "Who would you like to do the honors— you or me—your choice?"

Chapter 60

At precisely two p.m., Special Agent Frankie Banks knocked on the door of Jack and Madison's hotel room. The living area of their suite included a beige love seat and a glass-topped table. Its layout was generous in size and gave them ample room to sit comfortably.

"I was a little surprised to receive your call," she told them bluntly. "To be perfectly frank, Dr. Wyatt, I got the impression from our first meeting that you and Dr. Shaw weren't comfortable discussing matters outside the medical aspects of the cases with me. Now that things appear to be resolved, I'm left wondering why you reached out. I can only assume something's changed." Removing her spiral notebook and pen from her bag, she asked, "Am I correct in my assumption?"

"We've come across new information that we feel compelled to bring to the attention of the authorities," Jack said.

A casual smile came to her face when she said, "I'd very much like to hear all about it."

Madison said, "For the past few years, a number of Marsh employees have participated in a book club. A smaller group within the club decided to try their hands at writing and began exchanging their work to be critiqued by the other members. This group still exists and was composed of eleven members until a couple of weeks ago." She paused and added, "Now, there are nine."

Banks instantly lifted her eyes from her notebook. Her brow was furrowed.

"Dr. Shaw, are you about to tell me that these eleven individuals were the Marsh employees you recently treated at Georgetown Infirmary?"

"I'm afraid so," Madison answered.

"I'D LOVE to hear how you managed to find that out."

Madison and Jack then spent a few minutes explaining to Frankie how they had come to learn about the writing group and their submissions.

"You mentioned that Lori sent you the submissions a few weeks ago. Why did you suddenly get the urge to have a look at them this morning?"

"Other than things having been pretty hectic it didn't occur to me they could be important. It was probably just a mental hiccup."

"I see," Frankie said, unable to hold back a grin.

"Before I continue, may I ask you a couple of questions?"

"Of course,"

"The first time we spoke, you mentioned you were looking into two murders that occurred about a year ago near Newport News, Virginia. You also mentioned that the investigation brought you to the front door of Marsh Technologies."

"Right on both accounts, Dr. Shaw.

"By any chance did the murders involve twin brothers, and were they employed by Marsh's nuclear-powered submarine division as engineers?"

Letting out a breath, she finished making a note, leaned back, and interlaced her fingers. Her eyes moved over their faces.

"Okay, Doctors. Why don't you tell me just what you think you know?"

"John Winkler's submission was the first three chapters and a short summary of a novel he was supposedly working on. Both Dr. Wyatt and I think you should read it."

"I'd be happy to, but to save time, and for the purposes of this meeting, why don't I just ask you a few questions about his submission?"

"That would be fine."

"To begin with, how did he depict their deaths?" she inquired.

"They were killed in their sleep when their cabin blew up from a gas leak. Winkler portrays it as intentional. The main character is also a naval engineer and is employed by the same U.S. defense contractor that the twins are. While they worked in Newport News, he was assigned to the corporate headquarters in Washington, DC. Winkler paints him as a gifted expert in computer technology."

Jack said, "As an aside, while we were seeing John as a patient, we spoke with his wife several times. She was quite proud of him and mentioned on more than one occasion that he had an incredible God-given talent in the area of computer technology."

"So you're theorizing Winkler's book was more autobiographical than a work of fiction."

"That's what we suspect" Jack said. "There were several other interesting plot points, but the major one was that the engineer becomes suspicious that the twin brothers were heavily involved in an espionage ring. It was that involvement that resulted in their assassination. As I said, there are more details, but I think you've heard enough to understand our concerns. I'll email you Winkler's document so you can review it in detail."

"Thanks. I'll look forward to having a look at it. What I'm trying to understand is why Winkler would create a manuscript like that and then send it to ten of his colleagues."

"We can only guess, but since John survived the illness, that's a question you can ask him directly," Madison answered.

"Let me ask you a hypothetical question. I think all three of us are well aware that there's a possibility that these individuals were intentionally poisoned. From a medical standpoint, if they were victims of a crime, how do you think it could've happened?"

Jack responded, "Our best guess is by direct contact through the skin."

"Is there anything in their medical records that even hints at that?"

Jack and Madison hadn't talked about discussing the healing lesions on the patient's fingertips with Banks, nor had they considered the possibility she might ask. Hesitating briefly, Madison snuck an inquiring look Jack's way.

When he nodded in approval, she said, "Just before we started the treatment for heavy metal toxicity, we discovered that all the patients except one had tiny, barely noticeable, healing lesions on their fingertips. We think those lesions were caused by direct contact with the toxin, which further led us to believe the skin was the portal of entry."

"That's an interesting theory. You mentioned there was one exception."

"One patient had the lesions only on his index fingers," Madison responded.

"What medical significance would you attach to that?"

"Do you know what a hunter-pecker is, Special Agent Banks?" Madison asked.

"My aunt taught me how to type. She used the term frequently because my uncle could only type with his two index fingers," she said, as she began making another note. A few more seconds passed before she looked up with an impressed look on her face. "Applying the toxin to the keyboards of their computers—that was pretty clever of somebody."

"We thought so," Jack said."

"Who else knows about this?"

"We haven't shared the information with anybody except Dr. Hartzell."

"Do you know if she spoke to anybody about it?"

"If she did, she didn't mention it to us," Madison answered.

"So just to make sure I have this straight, for reasons and motives that are unclear, it seems that John Winkler felt the need to share his suspicions about a serious conspiracy involving Marsh with the other members of his writing group." Waiting for their response, Frankie glanced at each of them in turn.

"That's precisely the conclusion we came to," Madison answered. "The question is, how much of this would he be willing to divulge to the authorities after what he's just been through?"

"That's precisely what I'm going to do my damnedest to find out, Dr. Shaw."

"When we left DC a few weeks ago, John was the only one of the Marsh patients who was still struggling with cognitive impairment," Jack said. "As of now, we don't know how much he's improved, if at all."

Before Frankie could respond, Madison spoke up. "You'll excuse me for being so direct, Special Agent, but you haven't said very much. Do you have any concerns about what we've just shared with you?"

"I agree with you, Dr. Shaw—that was direct." A brief but telling pause ensued before she added, "I think the lives of the nine people who you and Dr. Wyatt fought like hell to save may still be at risk. What makes matters even worse is that tomorrow, they'll be leaving on what they see as a festive ten-day holiday. It's only natural that everybody will be in a joyful mood, secure in the belief that they've put a terrible experience behind them."

Frankie tucked her pad back into her bag and came to her feet.

"I'm going to ask both of you to not breathe a word of anything we've discussed here to anybody."

"Of course."

"I've got a lot to do between today and tomorrow. I can't thank you enough for making the decision to call me," she said as she started toward the door.

"If you don't mind us asking," Madison inquired in a reserved voice. "What are you going to do?"

"The same thing you and Dr. Wyatt did— I'm going to do everything in my power to make sure they live long and happy lives."

Chapter 61

The first call Frankie Banks made when she left Jack and Madison's hotel room was to Stuart Ortega, her supervisory special agent. With time hanging over their heads like a wobbling Sword of Damocles, they met within the hour to formulate a plan. At the conclusion of the meeting, they were in agreement that the FBI would provide security for the trip the Marsh patients were about to embark upon. They also concurred that, in an effort to avoid a firestorm of questions and demands for explanations from sources ranging from the physicians to everybody in the Marsh organization and perhaps even the press, they would implement their security protocol as discreetly as possible.

They considered the option of suggesting to March that the trip be canceled. After quite a bit of discussion it was Ortega's opinion that while their concerns were legitimate, they were also well short of a certainty. Suggesting the trip be canceled would undoubtedly create a flood of very challenging questions to answer. The result could be extremely damaging to the FBI's ongoing investigation. After a time, they finally agreed the best option was to provide appropriate security and allow the trip to proceed as planned.

They decided Frankie would remain with the group for the

entire ten-day trip, masquerading as a member of Marsh's public relations department along on the voyage to gather information for a story she was writing for the company magazine. The only ones at Marsh who were aware of the plan were the director of security and Erik Brickhill.

Accompanied by another FBI agent, Frankie arrived at Eaton Air, one of the more upscale executive jet operators at Ronald Regan National Airport's general aviation facility. Marsh operated four jets, with the flagship of the fleet being a palatially designed Airbus business jet that accommodated nineteen passengers and a crew of three.

The two agents had left themselves two hours to complete their security check before the anticipated departure time. They began by enlisting the assistance of one of TSA's canine explosive detection teams to complete a thorough sweep of the aircraft. They found nothing of concern. Frankie and her partner continued going through their entire checklist to make certain the aircraft was safe and secure for the flight to San Juan. In all, there were sixteen passengers. Eight were the Marsh patients and eight were their invited guests. With Anise planning on being out of town on her college tour, Nicole decided against making the trip without her.

As Frankie had planned, they completed the security sweep a full hour before the passengers were scheduled to begin arriving. She found a club chair inside the executive jet center to wait for the Marsh patients and their guests. She observed the first of the two pilots arriving. After spending a few minutes in the flight operations center, he exited the building, crossed the tarmac, and boarded the jet. Regularly flying globally, the aircraft was in the air almost every day and required eight pilots who worked on a rotating schedule.

A few minutes later, the passengers began to arrive. One of the executives from human resources was present to greet each of them. Once they were all present, she gathered them together in a nicely appointed conference room and took a few minutes to welcome them and review the itinerary for the entire ten-day trip. Frankie found herself paying particular attention to the guests of the Marsh patients.

Deciding to board before the group, she found a seat in a blue leather chair in the aft section of the jet. Once the meeting was concluded, the steward, Maxime, escorted the group aboard the aircraft, where they all settled in and were served a drink. Since the Marsh patients all had a few things in common, the atmosphere was relaxed, with several conversations taking place simultaneously. Frankie noticed the first officer come out of the flight deck, speak briefly with Maxime, and then exit the plane. She assumed he was attending to some last-minute details.

Thirty minutes later, the pilot made a brief announcement informing the passengers he'd been given his taxi instructions and that they'd be in the air and on their way to Puerto Rico in a few minutes. There were no ground delays, and ten minutes later they reached the threshold of the active runway and were cleared for takeoff. Once they reached their cruising altitude, the captain notified the group that they were free to move around the cabin. Frankie got up and took a self-guided tour through the opulent and spacious business jet.

"What do you think of her?" came a voice from behind her.

"Anybody who'd criticize a plane like this should have their sanity checked."

He chuckled. "My name's Maxime. I understand you're from public relations."

"That's me. I'm writing an article about the trip for the company magazine."

"Sounds like an assignment with nice benefits. May I get you something to drink?"

"No thanks. Talking about cushy assignments, it seems to me you have what most people would call a dream job."

"Two months after I was hired, I was still telling my friends and family to wake me up because I must be dreaming," Maxime responded. "The only problem with my job is you have to worry about every little detail. Like today. We were delayed about half an hour when we changed pilots. If that had happened on a commercial airliner, most of the passengers would be ecstatic that they'd only been delayed thirty minutes. We only have Marsh employees aboard this flight, so the pucker factor is considerably reduced. If this were the usual business flight where time is money or the Marsh elite were trying to impress some VIP...well, the expectations of perfection would go way up."

Since Frankie was unaware that there had been a last-minute crew change, she was struck by a guarded amount of concern.

"I didn't realize we had swapped out one of the pilots."

"Our first officer got sick and couldn't make the flight, so the captain arranged for the on-call pilot to replace him."

Frankie recalled seeing one of the pilots get off, but she hadn't paid much attention when he boarded again because he'd walked past her quickly and she'd only caught a glimpse of his back. She assumed he was the same pilot who had deplaned earlier.

"I saw him when he got off," she mentioned to Maxime. "I hope he wasn't seriously ill."

"He said he had a terrible migraine and that he didn't consider himself safe to fly."

"That seems a little strange."

"Not really. Safety always comes first."

"I mean, I saw him when he got off. I have two brothers who get terrible migraines and a couple of friends with the same problem. Whenever they have one, they look like they're on death's doorstep. They're pale, and their eyes are half-closed and watery. He looked fine to me."

"I guess migraines come in all varieties."

"The on-call pilot must live pretty close to have gotten here so quickly," she said.

"When they're called, they have a thirty-minute response time. There's no wiggle room."

Her uneasiness mounting, Frankie said, "I just had a thought. Maybe a good place to start the research for my article would be with the pilots. They'd probably love to be mentioned in it. Do you think they'd be willing to speak with me?"

"Do you mean now?"

"Sure."

With a grimace on his face, Maxime answered, "They're a little busy up there. It would probably be better if you caught up with them after we land."

"My brother's an airline pilot, and from what he tells me, I'll bet they're on autopilot, just monitoring things."

"Actually, there's an FAA regulation prohibiting any unauthorized individual to enter the flight deck during the operation of the aircraft."

She absently tapped at her lower lip. Plan A hadn't worked, leaving her deliberating whether her concern warranted blowing her cover to assure she'd be able to speak with the captain. Looking toward the front of the aircraft, she saw there was nobody between her and the door to the flight deck. She kept her back to the forward lounge and its occupants, continuing to face Maxime straight on. She slipped her wallet from her pocket and discreetly showed him her FBI credentials."

"I'm Special Agent Frankie Banks of the FBI, and I need to speak to the captain on an urgent matter."

"So the whole public relations thing and writing an article—"

"Maxime, I mean right now."

"I feel a heart attack coming on."

"You'll be fine," she said, thinking to herself that he probably wouldn't be her first choice for the crew member she'd want in a crisis. He walked a few feet away, picked up a wall-mounted phone, and called the captain. As soon as he ended the call, he returned.

"The captain will speak with you." He took a few steps forward, tapped on the door, waited for a few seconds, and then opened it.

"Thank you," she said with a polite smile.

"You're welcome…I think."

Frankie wasted no time in moving onto the flight deck. She produced her FBI credentials and introduced herself to Captain Virgil Sealy and First Officer Todd Gerrard. Sealy was a strapping man with a strong jawline and a short, strapping neck who had been a corporate pilot for the past twenty-three years. His record as an aviator was unblemished.

"What's going on, Special Agent?" Sealy asked.

"Other than telling you I'm providing security for the passengers and this flight, I'm afraid I can't share much else with you."

"I'm ex-military. I'm not going to ask you a lot of questions. Obviously something's on your mind, so how can we help you?"

"You made a last-minute crew change. Mr. Gerrard didn't get on the aircraft until we were almost ready to taxi out."

"And you'd like to know why?" Sealy inquired.

"I sure would."

"In the first place, I've been flying with Todd for five years and have come to know him personally. I'm way beyond comfortable vouching for him."

"I'm relieved to hear that, sir, but I'm much more interested in learning about the pilot who was too ill to fly. How often have you flown with him?"

"Actually, I've never worked with him."

"Do you know him personally?"

"I've never met him. He just joined our team a few weeks ago, but my understanding is that his flying credentials are excellent. We went through the pre-flight checklist together, and he seemed to know what he was doing."

"Do you recall his name?"

"Seth Shore."

"Did he mention where he was or what he was doing before coming to work for Marsh?"

"He was pretty much all business. As I mentioned, we were going through a pre-departure checklist. There wasn't too much idle chatter going on."

"Maxime said he had a severe migraine."

"That's what he told me."

"Did he strike you as being ill?"

"I'm not a doctor, but I'd say he looked okay. I didn't realize anything was wrong until he told me he was too ill to fly."

"I realize you were only with him briefly, but did he say or do anything that struck you as odd or unusual?"

"Nope, nothing at all," Sealy said with certainty.

Frankie paused to consider the possibility that she was overreacting to the crew change. But as she looked around the flight deck, she suddenly changed her mind.

"I see you each have a flight case next to you," she said to Sealy. "They seem smaller than I remember."

"With the advent of what we call electronic flight bags, we don't need to carry reams of documents, charts, and books with us any longer, so our flight cases have become smaller."

"So you each carry only one?"

"That's correct."

"And you generally keep them right next to you?"

"That's the way the flight deck's designed," he answered. "If you don't mind me asking, why the big interest in our flight cases?"

"I was just wondering, if each of you generally brings one on board and they're sitting next to you then who does this one back here in the stowage area belong to?"

Chapter 62

The captain and Todd turned in their chairs and swiveled their heads as best as they could to look behind them. The flight went silent as they exchanged a perplexed look.

"I guess Shore left it here. He must have forgotten it, which is understandable, if he had a bad migraine," Sealy pointed out.

"He must be a pretty forgetful guy," she said, already studying the appearance of the flight case.

"Excuse me?"

"Well, not only did he leave his case here, but he also forgot to put his name on it. Would you mind if I take a look at it?"

"I'm getting the feeling you might think it's an explosive device."

"The thought crossed my mind," Frankie answered.

"Our protocol on the subject's quite clear. If we're suspicious we've identified a bomb, we're not supposed to handle it."

"Would that include if it's found on the flight deck? Because if it is an explosive device, wouldn't this be the last place we'd want it?"

"Should we declare an emergency, Virgil?" Todd was quick to ask.

"No, not yet, but let's check in with ATC and give them a heads up. For now, let's follow our onboard protocol for a suspected bomb."

Frankie suggested, "Let's see if we can speak to somebody with the TSA explosive detection team. I'd like to at least unzip the case and have a look inside."

"I'll save you the trouble," Sealy said. "I remember now that Shore had the case when he sat down. I saw him open it and then zip it closed. He wasn't exactly acting like somebody who thought they had a bomb sitting on their lap."

"What did he take out of the case?"

"Nothing as I recall, but I was a little busy reviewing our flight plan at the time. And as I said, he wasn't behaving like somebody who thought they were at risk of getting blown to kingdom come at any moment."

Slowly easing the zipper back, Frankie studied the inside of the case. Besides what looked like a large electronic tablet, she didn't see anything else. She decided against unzipping the other three compartments. She slowly slid her hand inside the case and ran her fingertips along the device's edges. It had the typical feel of an electronic tablet. Moving her hand gingerly, she eased her fingertips down the backside and her thumb along the front.

After a few seconds she noticed two worrisome things: The first was that the tablet felt surprisingly warm; the second was that it seemed to be attached to the sidewall of the case. She tried to slide her hand between the tablet and the spot where it was fixed, but she couldn't. Using her opposite hand, she ran it over the outside of case. Separate from the tablet and within the wall of the case was a second object. It was rectangular and approximately the size of a cell phone.

"You look worried," Sealy stated.

"Something's not right. I think we need to get this case off the flight deck right now. Where should I put it?"

Offering no objection to her suggestion, Sealy said, "I'd put it as close as possible to the aft emergency exit. It's located right next to the master bedroom suite. Once you get the case in the bedroom, cover it with plastic and then as many towels and pillows as you can. I'll tell Maxime to keep everybody away from there." He turned back to Todd. "I think we have enough now to declare an emergency. Get on the radio with ATC and tell them our situation and that we're diverting to the nearest airport." He stopped briefly to consider his next move. "As soon as we've chosen the best field, let's take a closer look at the smoke and fire checklists."

"Anything else before I move the case, Captain?"

"No, go ahead."

With all due care, Frankie picked up the leather case and left the flight deck. She spotted Maxime on the other side of the galley hanging up the phone. He gestured toward her to join him.

"I just spoke to the captain and got my marching orders. C'mon. I'll show you the way to the bedroom."

They walked through the forward lounge and then the conference area, making their way to the rear of the jet. The passengers were busy in conversation and paid little attention to them.

"This is the suite," he told her as he quickly opened the door. "You might as well put it on the bed." He watched as she carefully placed the case next to the pillows. He continued, "I'll find something plastic to cover it with, then we can use the blankets and pillows that are already in here to pile on top of it."

But before he took his first step toward the door, the room filled with a peculiar hissing sound. They both turned and set their gaze back on the bed. It was barely perceivable, but a wisp of smoke was rising from the top of the flight case.

Frankie's mind and body quickly became adrenalized. "Where's the nearest fire

extinguisher?"

Maxime was already breaking for the door. "It's right outside in the corridor."

"Hurry up."

Before either of them could say another word, the hissing suddenly became muted by a high-pitched crackling noise. Frankie felt her heart miss a beat.

"What the hell..." Maxime said in a voice that vibrated with angst as he ran out of the room, returning in a matter of seconds with the extinguisher.

"There's more smoke," she said as he pulled out the safety pin.

All of a sudden, there was an earsplitting pop. An instant later, the entire top of the bed, backboard, and back wall were ablaze. Maxime leveled the hose at the fire. With his hands shaking as if he'd been tossed into an ice bath, he managed to squeeze the lever down and dowse a large section of the inferno. A cloud of smoke began to fill the room.

The only thing preventing the room from being totally engulfed by flames was the FAA's strict requirement for the use of flame-retardant materials in every aspect of the interior construction and design of all aircraft.

Just then, a young man appeared at the door.

"My name's Chris. I'm a firefighter," he said calmly, moving forward and extending his hands for Maxime to pass him the extinguisher. "I'll take it from here," he said, fearing that within thirty seconds the entire contents of the can would be exhausted. With no hesitation, Maxime handed it to him. As opposed to the way he'd been operating the extinguisher, Chris sprayed the flames in a more strategic and controlled way to conserve the extinguishing agent and make it more effective in putting out the fire.

"Do you have any other extinguishers onboard?"

"We're under thirty passengers. The FAA only requires one, but there's supposed to be a smaller one on the flight deck."

"I've got to go easy on what's left of the agent in this extin-guisher, so I may need the one from the cockpit."

"I'll let the captain know," Maxime said. "I should go and move the passengers up front."

"When you can, bring me a portable oxygen tank and mask. I'm pretty sure I'm going to need them."

Frankie left the bedroom with Maxime and hightailed it back to the flight deck. A thin cloud of harsh-smelling smoke was beginning to fill the central portion of the cabin. The passengers were already starting to become panicked. She wondered what was taking the captain so long to deploy the emergency oxygen system. When she reentered the flight deck, both of the pilots had donned their masks.

"How bad is it?" Sealy asked, his voice only slightly muffled by his oxygen mask.

"The device ignited as soon as we got it into the bedroom and created a sizable fire. There's some smoke in the cabin, and it's getting worse. Maxime's moving the passengers up to the forward lounge. We have a firefighter aboard and he's taken charge of trying to put the fire out."

"We've already declared an emergency, and we're heading to the closest airport. Did you see any structural damage?"

"The device was incendiary, not explosive. I'm fairly certain there's no structural damage to the plane from the ignition, but I can't tell you how much damage the fire is causing."

"I need to know the instant it's out. If there's no hope of putting it out, I need to know that as well."

"What about oxygen for the passengers, Captain? The emergency masks haven't come down yet."

"That's because there's been no emergency depressurization, and I'm trying to wait as long as I can to manually deploy the supplemental oxygen masks. The supply only lasts for about thirteen minutes. Depressurization will get rid of the oxygen, but it will only suppress the fire—it won't put it out. The big problem with passenger oxygen is that those masks leak like hell, which means a lot of oxygen gets into the cabin. If the fire is spreading, the added oxygen can make the situation much worse."

"How long until we land?"

"We're descending into Myrtle Beach International now. We should be on the ground in about fourteen minutes. I'll do my best to control depressurization and airflow from the flight deck. If we get much more smoke in the cabin, I'll deploy the masks. Keep us informed."

"Will do. Maxime said you have a smaller extinguisher on the flight deck."

Sealy pointed to it on the wall behind him.

"Take it. In the end, I'm afraid the only thing that's going to matter is getting this plane on the ground and the passengers off as quickly as possible. If we can't get the fire out...well, it's not likely smoke inhalation's going to be an issue." He paused briefly before adding, "ATC has a pretty good fix on us in case we have to ditch. Don't forget we need constant updates as to the extent of the flames, smoke, and any visible damage to the structure of the plane."

Frankie left the flight deck and joined Maxime in the forward lounge, where all his energies were being exhausted trying desperately to keep the passengers informed and as calm as possible. Some were huddled together not saying anything, their lips moving in silent prayer; others were near hysterical and inconsolable. A few were attempting to use their cell phones to make what they must have feared would be the last call of their lives.

"I need everybody to stay as calm as possible," Maxime again announced to the group. "The calmer your breathing is, the better. Stay as close to the floor as you can."

"Why aren't there any oxygen masks?" one of the passenger's guests demanded to know.

"The captain doesn't want to add any oxygen to the cabin until he's certain the fire's completely out," Frankie said.

"Why isn't it out by now?" Gretchen demanded to know, her arm around Lori's shoulder, pulling her closer. "She's pregnant, for god's sake. She needs to be on oxygen for the baby."

"As soon as it's safe, the captain will deploy the oxygen masks. Right now, his only focus is getting us on the ground as quickly and as safely as possible," Maxime said, walking over to Frankie. "I'll see if I can find another portable tank and mask."

Frankie left the lounge briefly to bring Chris the extinguisher. Still fighting the flames, he was using the extinguisher sparingly. The smoke had thickened, and he was using the portable tank of oxygen Maxime had brought him.

"The captain wants a report," Frankie told him, feeling her first twinge of air hunger and the sudden urge to cough.

"At this point, I think the bigger problem's smoke inhalation. Tell him I think I can keep the fire contained for a few more minutes, but that's all the time he's got. I'm sure by now there has to be some damage to the fuselage from the fire. These people need oxygen. I can feel us descending, but he needs to deploy the emergency oxygen system and get us on the ground."

Chris was a complete professional who was not prone to getting flustered under pressure, but his frustration was mounting rapidly.

"The pilot knows that. I'm guessing we'll be landing in about ten minutes."

Having more trouble catching her breath, Frankie hurried forward to see if there was anything she could do to assist Maxime. Just in the short time she'd been gone, the smoke was thicker. Everybody was coughing, and some were beginning to gasp. She grabbed the phone from the wall.

"Captain, these folks aren't going to make it another ten minutes. The smoke's getting pretty bad. The firefighter said the fire's mostly under control, but he doubts he can do any better. He strongly recommends deploying the emergency oxygen masks."

Sealy had heard enough. He reached forward to override the emergency decompression function and manually deploy the supplemental oxygen system.

"Tell Maxime to make sure everybody has a mask on. Once that's done, get them in seats with their belts fastened. If this plane stays in one piece, we'll be down in eight minutes. Warn him quietly that it's still a possibility I'll have to set us down in the Atlantic." Frankie didn't like the sound of his voice. She suspected the possibility of a water landing was higher than he was letting on.

She found a seat and donned her mask. She didn't realize how short of breath she was until she inhaled a few lungfuls of oxygen-rich air. She couldn't remember a time that she felt such utter fear. She was pleased that she'd functioned well despite her near-palpable fright, but with each passing second, she couldn't help but wonder how she'd hold up if the plane wound up in the ocean.

Captain Sealy continued his descent into Myrtle Beach International. It was the closest airport with a runway of sufficient length to accommodate the jet. He'd been assured by the tower that all emergency services had been mobilized and that they were ready to assist in any way necessary. They assured him the surrounding airspace had been cleared for his emergency arrival.

Frankie gazed out the window just as the jet broke through the clouds. The shoreline instantly came into view. The high speed and sharp angle of the descent were steeper than she'd ever experienced on a commercial airliner. Every few seconds the jet wobbled and vibrated with extreme force, sending a flash of fear that penetrated to her marrow. Overwhelmed with terror, most of the passengers were still frantic and screamed each time the aircraft shuddered. Despite the panic level reaching redline, Maxime remained focused and undaunted in his efforts to keep the situation from deteriorating any further.

Frankie estimated they couldn't be more than a thousand feet off the ground. She closed her eyes and began counting back from fifty—doing anything she could to make the time pass more quickly and get them closer to the end of the runway. Another minute passed, and she felt the landing gear rumble down. She prayed they'd be on the ground before the aircraft blew apart in midair. The thick, pungent smoke further permeated the cabin, making it impossible for her to see more than a few feet in front of her. Nobody had checked on Chris for the past few minutes. She hoped against hope he was okay.

Maxime pulled off his mask. "Brace position," he yelled. "Feet on the floor, lean forward, and cross your arms in front of your chest."

All at once, the main gear jolted against the threshold of runway one-eight. A few seconds later, the nose gear followed. The rollout began down the centerline of the runway, but as the aircraft decelerated Captain Sealey encounter difficulty with his rudder control causing the plane to swerve from one side of the centerline to the other. With twenty thousand hours of experience under his belt, he kept control of the jet and brought it to an abrupt but safe stop fifty feet from the end of the asphalt.

Maxime and Frankie came to their feet immediately. Rushing forward, he opened the forward emergency escape exit. A few seconds later both Sealy and Gerrard appeared in the cabin and began assisting the passengers in the evacuation process. Several applauded and cheered the instant they saw the two pilots. From all the movies she'd seen with imperiled aircraft, she couldn't believe how well Sealy had landed the jet.

The plane was met by a fleet of fire engines, rescue vehicles, and police cruisers. The firefighters boarded the aircraft immediately and extinguished the remaining flames. Chris came forward and joined the other passengers, where he was given a huge hug by his wife. Several other members of the rescue team joined the group up front and assisted in getting them off the aircraft and well away from the crippled jet.

A local emergency room physician was on site to assist in triaging the patients. In view of the smoke inhalation and their recent illness, it was her recommendation that they all be transported to the local hospital for a complete pulmonary assessment. A few, including Frankie, refused, but the majority didn't protest the trip to the emergency room.

As expected, the area remained a scene of major commotion. Once Frankie been escorted to a safe area, she identified herself to one of the police officers, who arranged to get her a ride to one of the private jet terminals. Fifteen minutes later, she was sitting in Execuaire's private lounge sipping on a large tumbler of ice water. She was breathing without difficulty, and from a purely physical standpoint, she felt no adverse effects from her harrowing experience.

While she sat there bleary-eyed, her mind began going over the details of what had occurred. She was drained of every ounce of energy, but the relief she felt was overwhelming.

The first phone call she made was to the local FBI office. She realized it was the beginning of an investigation that would be the most challenging and comprehensive of her career. Her second call went to her colleagues in DC to get them started on locating the migraine-stricken pilot. She didn't think they'd have much trouble finding him, and she hoped it would be easy to persuade him to divulge everything he knew. She suspected that being formally arrested would turn him into a fount of information.

A few minutes passed, and Frankie was starting to feel the weight of her eyelids, when Sealy and Gerrard walked in.

She couldn't contain a smile. "Nice landing, Cap."

He grinned. "Todd landed the plane. I was too afraid."

"He's kidding," Todd was quick to say. "He set that jet down more gently than a butterfly with sore feet." He added with a grin, "But if you think our chief pilot will buy that bedtime story about me landing the plane and give me a raise, I'll swear that's exactly what happened."

She chuckled as Sealy sat down beside her.

"I guess I could ask you what the hell happened up there, Special Agent, but I don't expect you'd tell me."

"As much as I'd love to, you may have to wait until the story's on the six o'clock news."

"When are you heading back to Washington?"

"In a few hours."

"You're kidding."

"My supervising agent's sending a plane for me. To put it mildly, he'd like to debrief me in person as soon as possible. Any preliminary word on the condition of the passengers?"

"From what I heard, everybody should be okay," he said. "A few of them might need to be hospitalized for a day or two to be treated for smoke inhalation."

"I guess you'll be answering a bunch of questions yourself from the FAA in the weeks to come."

"I was supposed to go fly fishing out in Montana next week," he said, coming to his feet. "I'm pretty sure I'll be putting the trip on hold. I suspect our paths will cross again sometime in the future, Special Agent."

"I wouldn't be surprised."

"Todd and I both want to thank you for your help. I imagine things would have turned out much differently if you hadn't been aboard. You don't have to be psychic to realize what would've happened if that device had ignited on the flight deck."

"Fortunately, that's something we don't need to worry about," Frankie said.

"We've got a mountain of paperwork to get started on. We'll let you get some rest." She watched as they made their way out of the lounge.

Three hours later, Frankie was at thirty-one thousand feet on her way back to DC. With the immediate crisis behind her, she began to consider what the next best step in her investigation should be. She was becoming more convinced with each passing hour that Marsh had a hand in the attempted murder of everybody aboard the plane. John Winkler's submission to his book club had suggested that their elite leadership had knowledge of illegal events going on in Newport News. But Frankie still wasn't certain if they were directly involved or had simply turned their back to it. She assumed that was one of many questions she'd be looking into in the months to come.

After a few more minutes of weighing everything that had happened, the lingering shock from her brush with death finally caught up to her. Overcome with fatigue, she was no longer able to keep a straight thought in her head. Feeling heavy-eyed, she closed her eyes. A minute later, she was asleep.

Chapter 63

With a container of Hazelnut coffee in hand, Erik strolled into his office. He spotted Emelia Cruz, his personal assistant since the first day he reported for work, standing next to his desk setting his printed agenda for the day on his leather desk pad.

"Good morning," he said, immediately noting the glum look on her face, a unique departure from her usual upbeat persona.

"Have you heard?" she asked him.

"I guess that depends. What are you referring to?"

"Our company jet carrying the Marsh patients had to make an emergency landing in South Carolina yesterday afternoon. There was a fire on the plane."

He stopped in his tracks. "My God. Was anybody hurt?"

"I don't have a lot of information, but I heard a few of the employees and their guests had to be admitted to the local hospital because of smoke inhalation."

"Do you know how serious they are?"

"Supposedly, they're being discharged today or tomorrow."

"And the rest are okay?" he asked.

"That's what I was told."

"I assume they canceled the remainder of the trip."

She nodded. "We sent a charter for the others last night and they're already back in DC."

With his mind starting to do backflips, Erik moved toward his desk and sat down.

Resting his chin on his hand, he said, "Can you get Jim Eiger on the phone for me, please."

"Actually, I saw him when I came into work. I'm pretty sure he's down in the trustees' office."

Jack came to his feet, marched out of his office, and walked down the hall. The door to the trustees' office was open. Jim was sitting at a small glass conference table with several documents in front of him.

A member of Marsh's board of directors for eleven years, he had been the one to spearhead the initiative to recruit Erik. The two of them hit it off immediately and over the years had remained good friends. Gruff at times, Jim rarely stood on ceremony, nor did he warmly embrace the necessity of being politically correct. Detailed oriented, quick on the uptake, and well informed, he took his position more seriously than most of his fellow board members.

Erik rapped on the door a couple of times and walked into the office as Jim waved him forward.

"I didn't know you came to work this early," he joked, leading Erik to suspect he hadn't heard about the incident involving the company jet.

He walked over to the table, took the seat across from him, and briefed him on what had happened. He wasn't surprised to see the color practically drain from his face.

"Thank God, they're all safe."

"My father was the smartest man I ever knew and only gave me advice on rare occasions," Erik said. "But I learned at an early age that when he did, the smart move was to embrace what he told me. The most important thing he ever advised me was to never do anything that would make me think less of myself for the rest of my life."

From the fretful expression that instantly landed on his face, Erik had no doubt Jim knew exactly what was on his mind. After tapping his lips for a few seconds, Jim got up and slowly walked over to the door and quietly closed it.

"I may not be the sharpest knife in the drawer, but I think I have a pretty good idea why you're here," he said, on his way back.

"Good, because I have a question or two I'd like to ask you."

He retook his seat and cleared his throat. "Every bone in my body is telling me not to discuss this with you," he said, as his eyes dropped away. "You have no idea where this information could lead you, Erik."

"I'm more than willing to take that chance."

"I'll tell you what I think I know, but it's quite possible it's not the entire story. I'm not going to try and extract any promises from you regarding what you're going to do with the information."

"Are you directly involved in any of this, Jim?" he asked him flatly.

"No, I'm not, but that doesn't mean my speaking to you about this…this situation won't spell disaster for me as well as you."

"The second most important piece of advice I got from my father was that it's never too late to do the right thing."

"It's funny you should mention that because I've been reminding myself of that nugget of wisdom every day for the past several weeks."

———

FIFTEEN MINUTES later their conversation was over and Erik had returned to his office. Over the past weekend, he'd given considerable thought to tendering his resignation as CEO of Marsh Technologies. At first, it was just a fleeting idea, but by Sunday evening he'd become convinced that moving on was an option that deserved his most serious consideration. If Erik was anything, he was a realist. He understood making a change of such proportions could turn out to be considerably more complicated than a polite parting of the ways.

He reached for his cell phone and placed a call to his longtime friend, Cal Blackwell.

"Hi, Erik. It's good hearing from you. How are you?"

"I'm okay."

"If you're going to invite me to go bouldering with you again, I'm not sure I've recovered from our last outing to Morgan Run. I'm still massaging myself in places I didn't know had muscles."

"I'm afraid this is a business call, Cal."

"While I'm flattered you'd think of me, but I'm a blue-collar criminal defense attorney, not one of your high-powered corporate guys."

"I'm aware of that," Erik said in a monotone.

"I see. How can I help?"

Taking in a lungful of air, he held it for a couple of seconds before exhaling. "I'd like you to arrange a meeting with you, me, and the FBI."

Following a measured silence, Cal said, "Okay, but I think it would be advisable for the two of us to sit down and discuss the problem before we walk into a meeting like that."

"You name the time and place," Erik said, barely able to push the words past the back of his throat.

"Can you be in my office tomorrow morning at ten?"

"Yes, I can."

"Good. If there's any material you'd like me to take a look at, bring it with you."

"I will. Thanks, Cal. I'll see you at ten."

"And one other thing— I don't know if you've been talking to anybody about this matter, but if you have, it stops right now."

"I understand."

"Listen, Erik. I obviously don't have the first clue as to what's going on, but I can tell you that oftentimes, from a legal standpoint, it's not nearly as bad as it seems.

"I hope that turns out to be the case. Thanks again. I'll see you tomorrow."

Despite Cal's encouraging words, Erik suspected his problem could easily turn out to be every bit as disastrous as he feared.

Chapter 64

At ten minutes to ten, Jack walked into the plush law offices of Welman, Schrager, and Delaney. As opposed to most of the venerable, carriage trade law firms in the Washington area, WSD Legal had only been in existence for forty years. But owing to their skill as investigators and litigators, the group was now counted amongst the best criminal defense firms in DC.

A couple of minutes after Erik had been escorted into the firm's conference room, Cal came into the room, walked over to the far side, and adjusted the thermostat.

"I don't know why the hell they insist on keeping it so damn warm in here. Can we get you something to drink?" he asked as he took the seat across from him and tossed his yellow legal pad down in front of him.

"I'm fine. Thanks."

"I'll skip most of the usual formalities, but I would like to mention a couple of things. After I've heard what you have to say, I'm going to lay out your options as I see them along with my recommendations. Should you decide to proceed with a meeting with the FBI, my main job's going to be to prep you in such a way as to make sure you don't say anything that could possibly implicate you in something illegal."

"Understood."

"Good. So why don't you begin by telling me how you came across this information that you'd like to share with the FBI."

"A lot of it, I figured out on my own by various means, and some of it came from a conversation I had with one of our board members."

"Did you approach him or her or was it the other way around?"

"I went to him. We've always had a close relationship and I suspected if anybody would be willing and able to enlighten me, it would be him."

"And was he?"

"Yes, he was."

"Okay," Cal said, picking up his pen. "We can talk more about that after you tell me the substance of why you're interested in speaking to the FBI."

"A few weeks ago, Everett Warren, the chairman of our board, came to see me. He advised me that Marsh was facing an unprecedented crisis and that he needed my help. Because I had no idea what he was talking about, I was more than a little surprised by his request. I took for granted he was sitting across from me because he wanted to bring me up to speed on a new problem. As it turned out, my assumption couldn't have been further from the truth, because all he told me was that the problem began a year ago and involved our facility in Newport News. He then informed me a consultant he had engaged would be contacting me in the next few days to fully brief me."

"You're the CEO. That sounds a little strange."

"I thought the same thing, but nevertheless, it's exactly what happened. It was obvious he was resolute about not discussing the situation with me, so I saw no reason to press the point. I decided to sit tight and wait for this…this consultant to contact me."

"And did that happen?" Cal inquired.

"Yes. A few days later a woman showed up uninvited at the restaurant where I was having lunch. She sat down at my table, identified herself as Regan, and told me she was working with the government to help Marsh deal with a major crisis. To my surprise again, she too chose not to share many of the details with me."

"What did she tell you?"

"She wanted to share with me that Marsh had gotten themselves into deep trouble, and that she'd been engaged to deal with the problem. She then may it crystal clear that my only responsibility in the matter would be to keep her informed."

"Of what?"

"She didn't say. She simply advised me she'd have a number of questions for me in the next week or so and that she expected I'd make myself immediately available to respond to her inquiries."

"Did she make contact with you again?"

"I spoke with her on two additional occasions. For reasons I didn't understand, she was quite interested in the Marsh patients and concerned the physician consultants who'd joined the team might create a problem."

"I'm not sure I understand. What kind of problem?"

"Drs. Shaw and Wyatt are quite well known nationally. She was quite concerned their presence would attract unwanted media attention. She also wanted my assurances that Dr. Hartzell, the physician employed by Marsh who was leading the physician group, could be relied upon to be a team player. The third and last time I saw her she told me her work was done and that I'd never hear from her again."

"What about the crisis she was engaged to deal with?"

"Again, she was vague, but I got the impression the crisis still existed."

"Okay, back to the board chair for a moment. I assume he didn't inform you that there was anything illegal going on."

"Not in so many words."

"I'm a little confused. If he didn't tell you anything and this woman who showed up at your lunch table was equally elusive, what's the nature of the information that you're so anxious to share with the FBI?"

"I suspect the federal government and Marsh conspired to cover up several felonies, including murder, and did their best to see to it that the eleven employees recently hospitalized at the Georgetown Infirmary would never leave the hospital."

Cal sat there in silence as a look of disbelief flashed to his face. He got up and walked over to a coffee maker that sat on a mahogany console table.

"Do you have any evidence to support that incredible accusation?"

"A little over a year ago our director of operations at our Newport News ship-building facility discovered two of our employees were stealing classified production documents and selling them to a foreign government. The two men were brothers and employed as marine engineers working on nuclear submarines. He also found out there was a third person involved in the conspiracy who turned out to be employed by GBA Systems, one of our sub-contractors."

Jim finished stirring in the third packet of artificial sweetener and then returned to his chair.

"You're talking about treasonous activity that would be a clear violation of the Espionage Act. I assume the director of the Newport New facility notified the FBI and Marsh's highest-ranking executives here in Washington."

"It's my understanding that he didn't."

"Are you implying that these espionage activities are still going on?"

"No, because two weeks after he discovered what was going on the two Marsh engineers were killed in a massive gas explosion that took place in their cabin. Whether the explosion was an accident or not is still under investigation."

"What about the third conspirator?"

"A few days later he went crabbing on the Hampton River and was never seen again."

Cal folded his burly arms in front of his torso. "Are you're suggesting that instead of following lawful procedures in a suspected treason and espionage case, this director attempted to cover-up the entire thing?"

"I'm afraid that's not what happened. I think as soon as he knew about the espionage activities, he reported the matter to the government. I believe his first choice was to follow a lawful pathway but the government representative, for his own purposes, had other ideas."

"What are you suggesting, Erik?"

"I'm suggesting the government very likely had a hand in every illegal thing that happened in Newport News and here in Washington."

"Why would the government see the need to go to such lengths to cover-up what happened. It's not as if our country's never been the victim of an espionage ring." Spinning his wedding ring, he added, "There has to be more to the story."

"Two and a half years ago, Marsh added *GBA Systems* to our list of subcontractors. Obviously, when you consider the number and size of the defense contracts we hold, that's hardly an unusual event, and unless there was a specific reason, would raise no eyebrows."

"If what you say is so, what's so special about GBA Systems?"

"A few things. Last night, I took a look at the subcontractor application they submitted to us. It was a little difficult to connect the dots, but I'd say there's pretty good evidence that we knowingly signed off on the subcontractor agreement full well with the knowledge that GBA's cybersecurity systems failed to meet required government standards."

"Why would Marsh take such a foolish risk?" Cal was quick to ask.

"Does the name Kennon Baich mean anything to you?"

Cal Interlocked his fingers behind his neck. "Only that he's the president of the United State's brother."

"I have strong reason to believe Baich has a considerable financial interest GBA Systems that is very well camouflaged. Apparently, he used his family clout and undo pressure to coerce Marsh into using GBA as one of our subcontractors. The end result was two enormously profitable contracts."

"And in return Kennon would use his leverage with the president to assure Marsh would be awarded a steady stream of defense contracts?"

"I have no evidence to suggest that's true," Erik answered with conviction.

"Even so, all of this begs the obvious question: Why in perdition would Marsh, an enormously successful corporation with an immaculate reputation, become involved in this illegal cover-up?"

"Because if they didn't and all the information regarding Baich's association with GBA Systems including the espionage committed by one of its employees became public, the resulting scandal would rock the country. Marsh would be accused of a quid-pro-quo relationship with the president's brother along with committing a long list of felonies including murder. For all intents and purposes, it would spell the end of Marsh Technologies."

"But you insist that a quid-pro-quo relationship truly didn't exist?"

"I don't think it did, but what's the difference? The accusation's as bad as the deed. Once all of this became public, Marsh would never again be awarded a defense contract. It would obviously spell the end of their company."

"Most of what you're telling me happened at least a year ago, but you said there have been other illegal activities here in DC recently. I'd like to hear about that."

Erik took the next forty minutes briefing Cal on the events of the past two months. He began with John Winkler's report and his meeting with Oren Severin. He then took him through the strange circumstances of the Marsh employees near fatal illness, summing up by recounting the events of the fire that occurred on the company's jet.

When he was finished, Cal got up, and again walked over to the coffee machine, this time making himself a decaffeinated mug of coffee.

"From a legal standpoint, do you know the difference between hearsay and legitimate evidence that would be admissible in a court of law?"

"I'm not in court, Cal. I have certain information that I'd like to make the FBI aware of. As I said earlier, a lot of it is circumstantial or the product of deductive reasoning. The point is that what the FBI does with that information is entirely up to them."

"You can count on them asking you specifically how you got your information."

"I've formulated some theories. If they can be verified, they'd almost certainly have enormous implications." Slowly shaking his head, Erik went on to say, "Maybe I should've had the courage to come forward with them sooner, but I'm not going to push anybody I believe to be innocent off of a ledge."

"I can't guarantee that'll work."

"It better because I don't have a plan B, and I won't be able to live with myself if I sit back intimidated and silent, pretending none of this ever happened."

Cal tossed his pen on the table.

"There have been a lot of good people who have gone to various government agencies

with the best of intentions. Sometimes, they were motivated by ill-conceived guilt. Maybe they viewed themselves as good Samaritans, conquering heroes, or, perhaps, even martyrs. But for a host of reasons things simply didn't turn out the way they thought they would."

"My mind's made up, Cal. I'm prepared to take that risk."

"As I was about to say, for me to sit here and try to talk you out of going to the FBI would be about as productive as shouting at the rain. But, as I mentioned earlier, if this is the minefield you choose to cross, it's my job to get you to the other side legally unscathed. There are steps we can take from a procedural standpoint to help guarantee that," Cal explained. "What I'd like to do before we set up this interview with the FBI is meet again so we can go over in extreme detail what I'd like you to say, how to phrase it, and what topics you should stay the hell away from."

"I'll make myself available whenever you say."

"How about Thursday, same time."

"I'll be here," Erik said, rising to his feet.

Cal escorted Erik out of the office and to the elevator. "This is an interesting first step you've taken—I'll give you that."

"I'll just take them one at a time. I've never been one to romance the truth or be irrationally optimistic, but if I have anything to say about it there are some unconscionable people out there who better start lawyering up. I'll see you Thursday."

Chapter 65

After a long day of doing nothing, Regan had dinner with her new love interest. She had already assumed her usual spot in the corner of the couch under a lightweight wool blanket when Alec strolled into the family room with two wine glasses and the bottle of pinot.

"I'm glad to see you're awake," he said. "I figured you'd be out cold by now."

"I'm pretty tired but I think I have another couple of hours in me before I crash."

"What's the chance of your butt getting dragged out of bed tonight by some dimwit your boss never should have hired in the first place begging you to come into the office to help them untangle some mess they created."

"Have a little faith. My plan is to be unreachable until seven a.m. tomorrow."

"That I'd like to see," he said, setting the bottle of wine and the glasses down on the end table.

"Aren't you going to open the bottle?" she asked without taking her eyes off the television. After a few seconds, when he didn't respond, she looked up at him. He had taken a few steps to his right and was now standing six feet away with a semiautomatic handgun leveled squarely at her chest.

"C'mon, Alec. I know the branzino I made for dinner wasn't great, but I think you may be overreacting."

"You really screwed up your last op, Regan. Too many people know about it, and they're not inclined to look the other way. But I'm glad to see you haven't lost your sense of humor."

"And here I thought they'd give me a mulligan." With a lazy shake of her head, she added, "Knowing how unoriginal Sol can be, I was kind of expecting something like this."

"I thought you'd be begging for your life. I'm sorry about this, but if anybody would understand, it should be you."

"What are you going to tell me next? It's not personal—it's only business?" With a whimsical snicker, she continued, "A trust-fund baby from Canada and a very successful day trader? C'mon, Alec. When you come up with a cover story, you should at least try to create one that's got some panache and not so easy to check out. Did you really think I wouldn't find out who you really are? Your fingerprints are all over this place." She wagged her index finger at him. "You should have stayed in the military and not become involved in work you clearly have no aptitude for."

"I'm not sure you're in a suitable position to criticize how I do my job." His hand had dropped a bit, the working end of his handgun now pointing more toward the floor.

"Did you even check my condo to see if I had a surveillance system? "For God's sake, Alec, I watched you after dinner when you went in the bedroom to check the clip in your Astra."

"That's smart, but maybe you should have done something about it then."

"You might be right, but I don't think it matters."

"Really? Why's that?" he asked.

"Because I'll be vanished and gone, and you'll be dead."

A look of surprise suddenly rushed to his face. He yanked the gun up to right his aim, but he was too late, and Regan knew it.

The volume on the television wasn't particularly loud, but it didn't matter. The silencer she had placed on the Beretta M9 that she held under the blanket did a nice job of suppressing the crack of the three shots she fired directly into his chest. The impact of the rounds sent him backward for a single long step before he collapsed and came to rest in a spread-eagle position on her throw rug.

She sighed and kicked off the blanket. Keeping the handgun pointed directly at him, she came to her feet in time to see him gasp his last agonal breath. The first thing she did was look around for his weapon. She spotted it about five feet from his outstretched lifeless hand. Strolling to his side, she kneeled down beside him and felt for a carotid pulse. There was none. She glanced at his eyes and noted his pupils were already beginning to dilate. Taking a moment, she examined the three tightly grouped entrance wounds in his central chest. Considering that she'd fired her weapon from beneath a blanket, she was pleased with the accuracy of the rounds, although she expected no less of herself.

Leaving him exactly where he'd fallen, Regan made her way into the master bedroom and stepped into her walk-in closet. In the back corner there was a dresser that held only a few bulky sweaters, which allowed her to slide it easily across the wood floor to expose her drop safe. Once she had it open, she removed three passports, ten thousand dollars in cash, and several government IDs and credit cards with various identities. Over the years she'd spent many hours planning for her hasty departure from the United States, if the situation ever called for it. She couldn't help but smile inwardly, imagining Sol sitting by his phone waiting for Alec's call confirming the problem of Regan Cullen had been taken care of.

She had a safe studio apartment about fifty miles away where she'd spend a few hours changing her appearance and making the final arrangements to leave the country. Once that part of her exit strategy was complete, her next stop would be Philadelphia International Airport and then on to New Zealand. She had no idea how long she'd stay there, but a part of her had always wanted to live there. Having more than enough assets to live comfortably for the rest of her life without ever working again, she found the idea of moving around a bit quite appealing.

She packed everything she needed for her immediate requirements in a carry-on and headed for the front door. Just as she was about to leave, she took one final look through the bay window at the Washington Wharf. She knew it was the last time she'd be able to enjoy the vista, but she'd had a long run, and there was a big part of her that was actually pleased with the way the evening had gone. Reveling in the prospect of beginning her new life, she took a final look at Alec, and then casually walked out of her condominium for the last time.

Chapter 66

Everett Warren finished packing his preferred leather suitcase, grabbed his cell phone, cash, and wallet from the top of his dresser, and proceeded to descend the spiral staircase of his six-bedroom house in Great Falls, Virginia. His wife, Amy, was waiting for him in their expansive marble entranceway. They had been married for ten years, which was longer than his first two marriages combined.

"Ready to go?" she asked him.

"I passed ready a week ago."

"You love our place in Alaska. Enjoy the hunting and fishing and try your best to unwind."

"Thanks. I'll certainly give it a try."

"Are you sure you don't want some company? I packed a bag just in case."

"It's pretty cold on the Kenai Peninsula this time of year. And since you're kind of an indoor girl, you'll be better off staying here."

"Whatever you say." It was the response he expected and was used to hearing, so he forced a tight smile to his face and walked out the front door, where Claude was waiting for him.

"Good morning, Mr. Warren," he said, taking his bag.

"Good morning."

"It's a beautiful day to fly, sir."

He absently gazed overhead. "So it is," He'd just called his pilot a few minutes ago. The company jet was fueled, pre-flighted, and ready to take him on the six-hour flight to Anchorage.

They walked down the cobblestone pathway to the Maybach. Just as Claude was about to open the door for him, a black Ford sedan pulled up behind the limousine. Frankie Banks got out from behind the wheel and approached him.

"Good morning, Mr. Warren. I'm Special Agent Banks," she said, producing her identification. "We'd like to speak with you at our offices. I'd appreciate it if you'd accompany me there."

"Would you excuse us a moment, Claude?"

"Of course, sir," he said, walking away.

"Now?"

"Yes, sir. Right now."

"Would you mind telling me what this is about?"

"I think it would be best if we had the entire conversation at our office."

"Do you have a warrant for my arrest?" he asked, trying to sound and appear as if her presence was nothing more than a nuisance and that she wasn't making him even a bit nervous.

"No, sir. I don't."

"In that case, I'm going to say no your request. I'll contact my attorney, and when I get back from my trip, we can discuss this again. Now, if you'll excuse me, Special Agent, I have a plane to catch."

She held up a folded document.

"Mr. Warren, I have a search warrant for your home that gives me the authority to detain you as long as necessary to complete the search."

The unworried look fell from his face.

"As a courtesy to you, I've arranged for our team to arrive here in fifteen minutes. In order to avoid an embarrassing scene, I'd suggest you reconsider your decision and accompany me to our offices now."

Banks looked around and then leaned in and said in a quiet

voice, "I think we both know it's an inevitability that we'll be taking this ride, so why don't we do it with as little fanfare as possible. If you'd like, you're of course welcome to call you attorney right now."

Warren looked toward his home and spotted Amy coming toward him. He raised his hand and motioned her to return to the house. She was close enough for him to see the mixture of worry and confusion in her eyes. She complied immediately with his request.

As he turned back to Banks, he felt a narrowing squeezing his throat. A wave of dread settled into his marrow as he realized the beginning of what he feared the most was now a reality.

Weakened by a sinking feeling of capitulation, he said, "My vehicle or yours, Special Agent?"

Chapter 67

ONE MONTH LATER

At Anise's request Jack and Madison had returned to DC to watch her compete in the finals of a citywide forensics tournament. They had flown in the day before and had met Anise for dinner. As far as they both could tell, she'd returned to her usual happy and chatty self.

Even though it was a blowy winter morning, Madison insisted they visit the Lincoln Memorial before picking up Anise and accompanying her to the tournament.

"I thought you only liked to visit the monument at night," Jack said.

"It's a different experience, but I love it almost as much during the day," she answered, staring up in awe at the details the sculptor, Daniel Chester French, had skillfully captured in creating Lincoln's hands.

"I can understand why you're so captivated by the Memorial," came a voice from behind them. "It's probably my favorite site in DC."

"Special Agent Banks, I almost didn't recognize you in your less formal attire," Madison kidded. "How are things going?"

"I'm deep in the throes of trying to figure out what to do with this giant Gordian knot you and Dr. Wyatt left me with," she said with a grin. "By the way, I think now would be as good a time as any for you guys to start calling me Frankie."

"We'll agree to Frankie if you say yes to Madison and Jack."

"Done."

"There's something I've wanted to ask you since you first introduced yourself to us," Madison said. "Is Frankie short for Francine, Francis, or Francesca?" Madison asked.

"None of the above. My parents loved Frankie, but they're not nickname people, so Frankie's my legal name."

"That never crossed my mind."

"Thanks for offering to take the time to speak with us," Jack said.

"If anybody deserves an update, it's you and Madison. I don't think I'm breaking any rules, though I may be bending a few. A lot of what we've learned has already made its way to the evening news. Even so, I'd appreciate it if you'd treat our conversation as off the record."

"Of course," Jack said.

"So here's the update. We're still gathering details. Some of what we know has come from John Winkler, but we only started talking to him a couple of weeks ago. After the accident, Dr. Hartzell and some of the other physicians were adamant about him needing more time to recuperate before being subjected to anything that could be stressful."

"Did he ever give you a specific reason why he sent the chapters and the cryptic outline of a novel to his fellow employees in the writing group?" Madison inquired.

"To tell you the truth, I think you two had it right. I'm not sure he knows why he did it. Evidently, he formally went to Oren Severin to report his concerns about the possibility of espionage activities at the Newport News facility. It wasn't an easy decision for him, and it was one that left him with a little buyer's remorse afterwards. The best I can figure is that he was looking for some kind of insurance policy. He wanted to remain anonymous, so he'd decided against going totally public. But at the same time, he wanted to drop some breadcrumbs that might connect the dots indirectly and lead to the truth, especially if anything happened to him. I'm not sure how much sense it all makes, but that was the best he could explain it."

"I guess the only thing that matters is that it made sense to him," Jack said, before shifting gears. "Were you able to find out anything about the adenovirus report we got from Fort Detrick?"

"I spoke with Dr. Benedict, who told me he never contacted any physician at the Infirmary about a viral culture result. So whoever called Dr. Hartzell was an imposter. From what we can determine, the specimens Dr. Hartzell sent did reach Derick's facility but mysteriously disappeared before they ever made it to the virology lab for analysis."

"So the obvious conclusion is that the written report was a complete fabrication," Madison said.

"I'm afraid so, obviously, by someone who didn't want to see any of the Georgetown Infirmary doctors questioning the diagnosis of viral encephalitis."

Jack asked, "Did you ever find out where the heavy metal poison came from?"

"One of the first things we did was assembled a team of special agents and lab technicians to try to figure that out. At the moment, they're leaning toward criminal elements with strong ties to Russia and China."

"Was our theory about the computer keyboards being the point of entry, correct?" he inquired.

"We were able to confirm that Marsh's office supply section delivered new keyboards to the eleven patients a few days before they started to become ill. We also have video surveillance of an unauthorized woman with a fake ID badge dressed in a Department of Office Inventory Management uniform delivering the keyboards. One of the security guards spoke with her but didn't suspect anything irregular was going on and never reported it. We've been trying to locate her, but so far, no luck."

"Unbelievable," Madison muttered. "The media's claiming that evidence exists that an illegal conspiracy including murder and influence peddling occurred and may have gone all the way to the White House."

"I can't be specific, but it's quite possible that in the coming months there will be hard evidence to confirm the allegation," Frankie said.

They slowly walked across the central chamber.

"If this governmental house of cards does get scattered to the wind by a stiff gust," Frankie continued, "hopefully, there won't be enough get-out-of-jail-free cards to protect those responsible." Halting momentarily, a disillusioned look appeared on her face. "The unfortunate truth is that the government often finds a way to do whatever's necessary to avoid being embarrassed. Unfortunately, there's usually ample room under the blanket of national security to protect select individuals from accountability. During my short career, I've seen some pretty unprincipled people avoid scrutiny because they were supposedly acting in the best interest of preserving our national security." With a modest shrug of her shoulders, she added, "I guess we'll just have to wait and see."

They continued to talk for another few minutes before wrapping things up.

"How much longer do you think you'll be working on this?" Jack asked.

"From the way things look now, I hope to be done before my retirement party," she answered with a smile. "How long will you be in DC?"

"Just through the weekend," Jack said.

"I should probably get going. If you guys need me for anything, give me a call. It's been a pleasure getting to know you both."

"The feeling's mutual," Madison said.

They watched as Frankie descended the steps and disappeared into a crowd of visitors.

"We should probably get going," Jack said.

Madison took him by the hand and gave him a quick kiss on his cheek.

"What was that for?"

"It's the recognition you deserve for being such a good man."

About Gary Birken, M.D.

When I first set pen to paper as a novelist, I was a busy full time pediatric surgeon. I completed eight years of surgical training at Ohio State University and Nationwide Children's Hospital and remain to this day an ardent Buckeyes fan. Upon completing my training, I relocated to South Florida and joined the medical staff of Joe DiMaggio Children's Hospital, where I served as the Surgeon-in-Chief.

Now that my schedule is more relaxed, I'm able to devote greater time to writing and getting more involved with my readers. My approach to story-writing has always been to utilize fiction not only as a means to entertain, but also to offer some insight into an interesting or controversial topic in medicine. I'm often asked by aspiring authors for suggestions as to the best way to get started. The best advice I can offer any individual who seriously want to write is to take the time to learn the craft of fiction writing, and then - read a lot and write a lot.

I am a member of the Mystery Writers of America and have had the opportunity of teaching writing at various conferences and other forums. I have also had the pleasure of serving as a panel member at the SleuthFest Conference. In addition to spending time with my family, including my ten grandchildren, I am a private pilot, and an avid tennis player. I also enjoy auditing university level courses and just hanging out with my English Setter, Eliza Doolittle. I hold a black belt in martial arts and frequently teach courses in women's self-defense.

facebook.com/GaryBirkenMD

instagram.com/garybirkenmd

Printed in Great Britain
by Amazon

55770362R00209